THE
SWEET DREAMS
BEAUTIFUL HAIR BOOK

You've seen it happen before: A girl with beautiful hair walks into the room, and everyone's head turns. You think, "I wish my hair was as shiny and bouncy and manageable as hers," but you don't know where to begin.

It's true that gorgeous hair doesn't just happen, but it doesn't have to take a lot of time and effort. All you need is know-how, and that's what this book provides: How to pick the shampoo and conditioner that's right for your type of hair and the cut and style that flatters your face. How to use the tools of the trade—from brush to blowdrier to curling wand. How to spark up your natural color and style your hair for day, night, or sports. And how to diagnose your hair problems like an expert.

The secrets of beautiful hair are all here. So if you want to turn a few heads, start by turning the page.

Bantam Sweet Dreams Specials

THE SWEET DREAMS LOVE BOOK
by Deidre S. Laiken and Alan J. Schneider
THE SWEET DREAMS BODY BOOK
by Julie Davis
THE SWEET DREAMS BEAUTIFUL HAIR BOOK
by Courtney DeWitt

The
Sweet Dreams
Beautiful
Hair Book

by Courtney DeWitt

Illustrations by Elaine Yabroudy

BANTAM BOOKS
TORONTO · NEW YORK · LONDON · SYDNEY

The best sources of information about applying the hair products described in this book are the manufacturers of those products. Always follow the manufacturers' directions exactly as they appear on the packages. If you have allergies, or think you may have allergies, you should check with your doctor *before* applying any preparation to your hair, and you should immediately stop using any product that causes irritation or discomfort.

RL 6, IL age 11 and up

THE SWEET DREAMS BEAUTIFUL HAIR BOOK: A GUIDE TO HAIR
CARE, CUTS, AND STYLES
A Bantam Book / June 1983

*Sweet Dreams and its associated logo are registered trademarks of Bantam
Books, Inc. Registered in U.S. Patent and Trademark Office
and elsewhere.*

Cover photo by Pat Hill
Book Design by David M. Nehila

ISBN 0-553-23375-0

Published simultaneously in the United States and Canada

PRINTED IN THE UNITED STATES OF AMERICA

0 9 8 7 6 5 4 3 2 1

To my family for their love and support

CONTENTS

The
Sweet Dreams
Beautiful
Hair Book

YOUR HAIR—DON'T FIGHT IT, FLAUNT IT!

*Straight, curly, fuzzy, snaggy, shaggy, ratty,
matty... fleecy, shining, gleaming, steaming, flaxen, waxen, knotted, polka-dotted,
twisted, beaded, braided, powdered,
flowered and confettied, bangled, tangled,
spangled and spaghettied... flow it, show
it, long as God can grow it, my hair.*

Hair is truly a natural wonder. It comes in all shades,
shapes, textures, and lengths. It responds to the envi-
ronment, reflects your overall health, and mirrors
your moods. If something isn't right in your life, your
hair, like a good friend, will let you know. Why then, do
so many people regard their hair as their worst enemy? They think it's too straight or too curly, too short
or too long. Either it lies too flat or it springs up in all the
wrong places. The color is too brassy or too dull.

The truth is, there's no such thing as perfect hair.
Everyone's hair has quirks, but that's what makes
it unique. The authors of the musical *Hair* had the
right idea. They recognized hair for what it is—your
crowning glory—no matter what form it takes or what
flaws it has.

The key to having beautiful hair is learning to live
with, and love, the kind you've got. You can perm it,
straighten it, color it, and cut it, but nothing will perma-

11

nently change the type of hair you were born with. It's yours for life. However, it can look fabulous or lackluster, depending upon the way you treat it.

Hair that behaves the way you want it to doesn't just happen. You have to work at it. It doesn't take much time or effort, but you do need a little know-how. And that's what this book is all about. You'll find everything from the basics of hair care—shampooing, brushing, and conditioning—to natural rinses that will spark up your hair color. There are sensational hairstyles for day, night, and sports, and super accessories that you can make yourself. You'll even learn how to diagnose your hair problems like an expert.

The more you know about your hair, the healthier and stronger you can make it—and the prettier you'll look. Just knowing that your hair looks its best and brightest will give you a great feeling— confidence in yourself. So stop fighting your hair and start flaunting it. All the tips and tricks you need are right here.

1

THE BASICS

How does your hair look right now? Is it full of bounce and body, or is it flat and flyaway? Does it shine as much as you'd like it to, or is it lifeless and dull? Is it easy to manage or hard to control? If your hair doesn't look as good as you think it should, chances are you're not giving it the care it needs. But before you can take steps to correct what's wrong, you have to understand what you're dealing with. Here are a few facts you should know about your hair.

Hair is made mostly of protein, called *keratin*. Each strand is composed of three layers: The outer portion is the *cuticle*, the middle part is the *cortex* and contains the pigment that gives your hair its color, and the heart of the hairshaft is the *medulla*. Hair is alive only at the root, which grows out of a tiny sac or *follicle* beneath the surface of the scalp. The hairshaft itself is dead; that's why it doesn't hurt to have your hair cut.

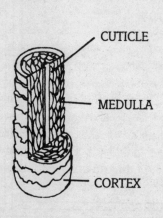

CUTICLE

MEDULLA

CORTEX

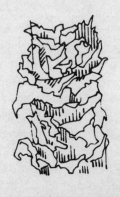

ROUGHED UP CUTICLE

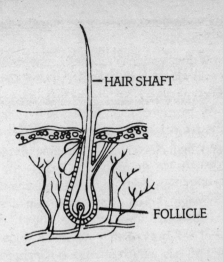

— HAIR SHAFT

FOLLICLE

If you looked at a strand of hair under a microscope, the outer layer would resemble shingles on a roof. Why? Because the cuticle is composed of overlapping cells. When these cells lie flat, your hair has a beautiful sheen. But if the cuticle has been roughed up by continual blowdrying or too much brushing, it will stick up and your hair won't look as glossy.

The life-span of any single hair on your head is two to six years. It's normal to shed about sixty to a hundred hairs per day, so don't be alarmed if some comes out when you comb or brush your hair.

The state of your hair is a direct reflection of your overall health. In fact, you might have noticed that when you're feeling under the weather, your hair tends to look droopy and lackluster. Healthy hair thrives on healthy habits. And that means a well-balanced diet full of protein and fresh fruits and vegetables—plus plenty of rest and exercise.

Shampoo—
Which One Is Right for You?

One of the nicest things you can do for your hair is to keep it sparkling clean. To do that, you need a good shampoo. No shampoo can change the type of hair you were born with, but it can make your hair easier to manage. A great shampoo doesn't have to be expensive. It should be strong enough to cleanse your hair of dirt, but not so harsh that it strips your hair of essential oils. Which shampoo is right for you? That depends on your hair type and texture. Other factors that are likely to influence your choice: whether you like using a liquid or a cream, the scent and color that appeal to you, and the kind of container the shampoo comes in—a bottle or a plastic tube. You'll probably have to try a few shampoos before you find one that suits you.

In general, the best way to judge a shampoo is by the way it makes your hair look and feel. Your hair should be shiny, bouncy, and manageable. If the shampoo you've been using irritates your scalp in any way, or if it dulls or dries out your hair or makes it too oily, switch to a different brand.

You'll find everything from eggs to milk to avocados in today's shampoos. The bottom line on fancy ingredients is that they won't do anything special for your hair; most of them go right down the drain during the final rinse. But if an ingredient such as honey appeals to you, or if you can't resist the sweet scent of strawberries, by all means use that shampoo. Just don't expect it to work wonders. Shampoos containing all-natural ingredients are good if you shampoo your hair every day because they're very mild and usually don't contain detergents.

Many shampoos are now pH balanced. The pH scale ranges from zero to fourteen, and the numbers refer to the acidity or alkalinity of the formula. Neutral pH is seven. Numbers lower than seven on the scale get gradually more acidic; numbers from seven to fourteen are progressively more alkaline. All hair is naturally acidic and falls between four and five on the scale. A pH-balanced shampoo is slighty acidic and attempts to match the natural pH balance of human hair. But no shampoo can match it exactly. To make any difference to your hair, the pH of a shampoo would have to be very high or low on the scale. An extremely alkaline formula would dull and dry out your hair. One with a high acid content wouldn't lather up enough to make you feel you were getting your hair thoroughly clean. Basically, a pH-balanced shampoo is very mild; it won't hurt your hair, but it won't have any special effect, either.

What Kind of Shampoo to Choose

Hair that gets heavy and greasy within a day of washing needs a shampoo made for oily hair or an oil-free formula. For hair that's dull and flyaway, is split or brittle, and snarls easily, a dry-hair shampoo with built-in conditioners is best. Castile-based shampoo and baby shampoo are also good for dry hair, because they're extra mild.

Silky, baby-fine hair that goes limp as soon as you walk out the door will get a boost from a shampoo formulated for "extra body." If your hair is both oily and fine, don't use a shampoo for oily hair; it will be too harsh. Also avoid using balsam-based shampoos or those containing heavy conditioners; either of those will make your hair too soft.

Wiry, coarse hair that has a tendency to frizz when the weather is damp will be easier to control if you use a protein-based shampoo.

For hair that retains body and shine for several days between shampoos, look for a normal-hair formula.

There are also hypoallergenic shampoos from which all allergy-reactive ingredients, such as fragrance, have been omitted. These shampoos are formulated for people who have sensitive skin (your scalp is skin) and are made for all hair types.

If you have dandruff, select a shampoo for your hair type—normal, dry, or oily—containing an anti-dandruff agent such as selenium sulfide or pyrithione. Dandruff shampoos can be drying, so use them only as often as necessary to control oiliness and flaking. If the problem persists, see a dermatologist.

Powdered dry shampoo can be helpful in a pinch, especially if you have long hair. You sprinkle it on, fluff it through your hair, and leave it on for a few minutes. Dust, dirt, and oil are whisked away when you brush it out. A dry shampoo is not a substitute for a regular shampoo because it doesn't get your hair really clean. Also, it can coat your hair with a dull film if it's not thoroughly removed, so make sure to wash your hair with a deep-cleaning shampoo as soon as you have time. Cornmeal makes a very good dry shampoo. Just dust it on your hair and massage it through for about five minutes. Then comb or brush it out.

Shampoo-stretching tip: If you're running low on shampoo, dilute it with an equal amount of water. It will still get your hair clean, and you won't have to go without washing your hair until you have time to buy more.

Shampoo How-To's

Even the best shampoo won't perform well unless you use it properly. If shampooing takes you only a few minutes, your hair probably shows it with masses of tangles or dull, limp-looking locks. It's worth spending a few extra minutes to do the job right. The payoff: hair that's shiny, swingy, superclean!

Here's the way to handle your hair when you wash it: with care. Imagine that it's a delicate piece of lace. You wouldn't pull or tug at a fragile fabric, would you? It might tear—and so will your hair if you don't treat it gently. Follow these simple steps and you're sure to get great results.

1. Brush your hair to remove tangles and loosen dirt and oil.

2. Wet your hair thoroughly with warm, *not hot*, water. (It's best to wash your hair in the shower. If you don't have one, you can buy a nozzle that attaches to

your bathtub faucet to make shampooing and rinsing easier.) Pour about one teaspoonful of shampoo (a little more if your hair is very long) into your palm. Rub your hands together to spread the shampoo, then apply it to your hair, starting at the top or sides of your head.

3. Using your fingertips, rub the shampoo lightly into your scalp to work up a good lather. Continue to work in the shampoo till you've covered every inch of your scalp. Pay special attention to hard-to-reach spots, like the nape (or back) of the neck, and areas where dirt and grime tend to collect, such as the hairline. Massage gently to avoid tangling or damaging your hair, and tilt your head back to avoid getting shampoo in your eyes.

4. After you've finished the scalp, work shampoo out to the ends by combing through your hair with your fingers. Take care not to scrunch up your hair in the process, or it may become matted. One lathering is enough unless your hair is very dirty.

5. Rinsing is the next and most important step. If you don't remove every last trace of shampoo, it can leave a dulling film on your hair and make it look lank and lifeless. Use lukewarm water for rinsing and make sure the spray hits your head from every angle. If you have long hair, you might want to divide it into sections while you're rinsing. You can also try bending over or lifting up the hair at the nape to remove suds that may be trapped there. Surprisingly, rinsing takes longer than shampooing.

A good rule of thumb: Rinse your hair twice as long as you think you should. Before you finish rinsing, run your hands through your hair—especially the area behind your ears—to make sure you've removed all the lather. Turn the tap to cool and rinse again to make your scalp tingle and to give your hair extra shine.

6. Next, apply conditioner. Leave it on for the time specified on the package label and rinse out thoroughly. (For complete how-to's, see page 26.)

7. Press your hair with your palms to remove excess water—never wring or twist it. Wrap your hair in a towel to blot up moisture, and pat dry. Don't rub vigorously; hair breakage may result.

8. Comb out your hair with a plastic comb that has blunt, widely spaced teeth. Start at the ends and work your way up to the top. Gently comb out snarls.

BRUSH UP

Brushing is a basic part of any hair-care routine. It keeps your hair shiny and healthy by distributing natural oils and dislodging surface dirt and dust that accumulate during the day. More bonuses: Brushing stimulates the scalp and is relaxing, too.

Brushing a hundred strokes a day might have been recommended in Grandma's day, but not anymore. Overbrushing can cause breakage and make your hair look greasy. About twenty-five strokes a day is all it takes to keep your hair shiny and manageable.

The Way to Brush

There's a right way and there's a wrong way to brush your hair. Don't tear at it with quick sharp strokes. A hurried brushing won't do your hair much good, and brushing too hard can even hurt it. To get the full ben-

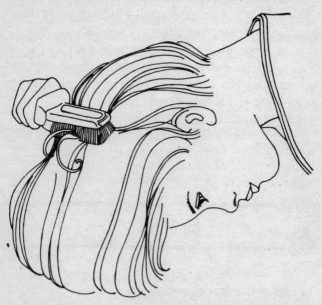

efit of brushing, bend from the waist and—starting at the nape of the neck—gently brush in a smooth lifting motion all the way out to the ends of the hair. This will distribute oils from your scalp to the oil-thirsty ends. If you encounter snarls, work them out gently with your fingers.

You can brush while you're listening to records or the radio. Or brush your hair while you're in bed.

Here's how: Lie on your stomach so that your head dangles over the edge of the bed and brush from nape to ends. You'll love the tingle it gives your scalp when you're done. When you're brushing to style your hair, stand or sit in an upright position and brush with long even strokes.

Words to the wise: Never brush wet hair. You might yank out healthy hair or cause split ends. Why? Your hair is more elastic when it's wet, and when stretched taut with a brush it can break easily.

Buy the Best Brush

Brushes come in all sizes and shapes. Bristles can be soft or stiff, natural or synthetic—or a combination of both. The tips should be blunt and rounded—never sharp. The type of brush you choose depends on how you want to use it and on the length and texture of your hair. In general, the thicker your hair, the stiffer the bristles should be.

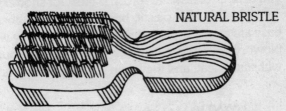

NATURAL BRISTLE

A soft, natural-bristle brush gives a nice polish to fine hair. For medium-textured hair, look for a brush with slightly firmer bristles—natural or synthetic. If your hair is thick and coarse, a stiff-bristled brush or combination brush is best because it will reach right down to the hair roots.

Before you buy a brush, run it down the inside of your arm; it shouldn't prick or scratch your skin. If a brush doesn't feel right on your arm, it won't feel right on your scalp.

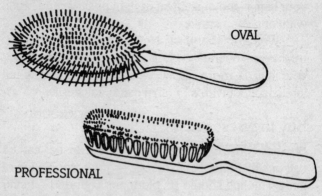

OVAL

PROFESSIONAL

What shape of brush should you choose? For long hair, a flat oval brush can't be beat because it covers the most territory in a single stroke. A slim, rectangular, "professional" brush is great for shorter hair.

Brushes with plastic bristles set in a rubberlike base are excellent for styling the hair, especially when blowdrying. They're lightweight, flexible, and built to withstand heat, and they won't damage damp hair.

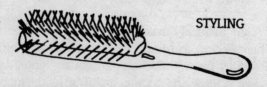

STYLING

Styling brushes range in size from about one inch to two and a half inches in diameter. For thick straight hair that's on the long side, a large flat styling brush works best. For wavy or curly hair, use a large round or half round brush, and for short fine hair use a small round model. Small round brushes are also good for styling bangs and layered hair.

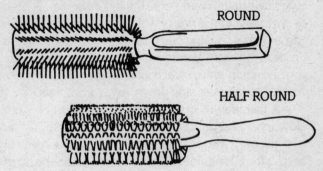

ROUND

HALF ROUND

To keep oily hair fresh between shampoos, try this trick: Cover the bristle end of your brush with a piece of gauze. Wind a rubber band around the brush at the base of the bristles to keep the gauze in place. Then brush your hair as usual. The gauze will absorb excess oil.

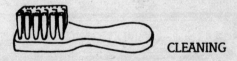

CLEANING

Keep It Clean

Wash your brush (and comb) every time you shampoo your hair. Otherwise, you'll be putting dirt back into clean hair. First remove old hairs from your brush. You can do this with a comb or a special cleaning brush—a short, squat, stiff-bristled brush you can buy at most drugstores. To wash your hairbrush, dunk the bristle end in warm sudsy water. You can use shampoo or a mild detergent in the wash water. Swirl the brush around until the dirt dissolves. A drop of ammonia in the water will help dissolve stubborn grime. Avoid soaking your brush—it can weaken the bristles and can destroy a wooden handle. Rinse your brush in warm water and shake off the excess water. Dry it bristle side down, away from heat.

A fast way to dry a styling brush: Turn on your blowdryer and direct a jet of air at the brush. If you take proper care of your brush, you can expect to keep it for a long time. Some natural-bristle brushes last for years.

Tip: Install a hanging grid in your bathroom to hold your blowdrier and other hair-care items. You can buy one in a store that sells housewares. Just plunk your hairbrush through a square of the grid so it's suspended handle side down. It will dry in a flash and always be within easy reach.

 ## CONDITIONING COUNTS

Conditioning is that extra step that can turn so-so hair into a glorious mane. A good conditioner will add body, bounce, and luster to your hair, and it will remove tangles, reduce static electricity, and tame the frizzies. If used on a regular basis, it can help prevent problems and keep your hair in top condition.

Who Needs It?

Everyone's hair needs to be conditioned. Normal wear and tear can take a toll. Blowdrying, hot rollers, perming, and straightening can rob hair of natural oils and ruffle up the cuticle so that your hair doesn't shine. Hot sun and cold wind are also enemies of healthy gleaming hair. For hair damaged by any one of these factors, there are two basic types of conditioners: instant and deep-penetrating.

An instant conditioner is a lightweight liquid containing ingredients such as balsam or protein to make the hair shinier, springier, easier to handle. It works by filling in the cracks and crevices in the hairshaft, and leaves a protective coating that lasts until your next shampoo. An instant conditioner is left on the hair for about two to five minutes, then rinsed out. Many shampoos now come with built-in instant conditioners.

A deep-penetrating conditioner does everything an instant one does—and more. It pampers and protects the hair, and helps repair damage by penetrating the hairshaft to restore lost moisture. Deep-penetrating conditioners are usually labeled for "dry, brittle, or damaged hair."

There are two kinds: rich cream conditioners and hot oil treatments. Both offer first aid to hair showing signs of abuse: lack of shine, split ends, dryness, and breakage. Most cream conditioners contain protein to help restore hair to its former glory. Depending on the type you use, a cream conditioner can be applied before or after shampooing. It's left on the hair for ten to thirty minutes (as specified on the package instructions), then rinsed out. It's important to rinse thoroughly because this type of conditioner can leave a residue that flakes off when you comb or brush your hair. For best results, apply the conditioner to your hair from roots to ends using a wide-tooth comb.

A hot oil treatment is another intensive conditioner that helps restore luster and manageability to extremely dry, brittle hair. It comes in a small plastic tube that's heated until lukewarm. It is then ready to be massaged into the hair and scalp. You can make your own hot oil treatment using a light vegetable oil such as safflower, sunflower, corn, olive, or almond oil (available at any health food store).

How to: Wash your hair and then towel it dry. Heat about three tablespoons of oil in a small saucepan (use less if your hair is short). Very important: Always test the temperature of the oil before you apply it to your hair. It should be warm—never hot. Hot oil can burn your hair and scalp. Comb the oil evenly through your hair using a wide-tooth comb. If your hair is dry only on the ends, apply the hot oil to the damaged portion of your hair, keeping the oil away from your scalp. Leave it on for twenty minutes, then wash your hair thoroughly to remove it, and condition as usual.

If your hair is naturally dry, give yourself a hot oil treatment every few weeks. If your hair's badly damaged, give yourself a hot oil treatment once or twice a week until the condition improves.

Products called "creme rinses" aren't really conditioners in the true sense. They are applied to freshly shampooed hair, left on for a few minutes, then rinsed out. Creme rinses soften the hair and make it sweet-smelling. They smooth out tangles and help tame flyaway hair, but they don't provide the protection that instant and deep-penetrating conditioners do. Avoid using creme rinses if you have fine hair.

Hairdressing creams, such as Alberto VO-5, which are left on the hair between shampoos, add shine to dry or dull hair and smooth down split ends, but they are only temporary measures.

Special note: To make any deep conditioner penetrate more effectively, wrap your hair in a warm wet towel after applying it, or cover your hair with a plastic bag. If the towel cools before it's time to rinse out the conditioner, replace it with another one or reheat it.

How to Choose and Use a Conditioner

The kind and amount of conditioner you should use depend on the type of hair you have and the condition it's in. If you have normal hair, you don't have to load it down with a heavy conditioner after every shampoo. Dry, damaged hair needs intensive conditioning. But in general, everyone should use a deep conditioner once a month to keep hair healthy and strong.

Here are some guidelines to help you choose the right conditioner and use it correctly.

• OILY HAIR Oily hair needs the least amount of conditioning because it has enough natural oil of its own. Use an oil-free conditioner once or twice a week if you need to. If your hair is very oily, concentrate conditioner on hair ends, taking care not to get it on your scalp.

- DRY HAIR For dry hair, conditioning is essential. Use an instant conditioner after every shampoo and a deep-penetrating conditioner once a month. For very dry hair, use a hot oil treatment.

- NORMAL HAIR If your hair snarls easily, try a shampoo and conditioner in one. If tangles aren't a problem, use an instant conditioner twice a week to keep your hair in perfect condition.

- FINE HAIR Use a light, body-building conditioner once or twice a week. If your hair is on the oily side, use an oil-free conditioner instead. Never use creme rinses or conditioners containing balsam— they may leave your hair too limp.

- COARSE OR CURLY HAIR A creme rinse or instant conditioner after every shampoo will make your hair more manageable. If your hair tends to be dry, use a deep conditioner every two to four weeks.

- DULL HAIR An instant conditioner used after every shampoo will make your hair glisten. Rinse again and again until you've removed all traces of conditioner. Too much conditioning might have caused your problem in the first place.

Sometimes conditioning can be too much of a good thing. If you use too much conditioner and don't rinse it all out, your hair will look drab and lifeless. Another side effect of overconditioning is that hair gets dirty faster. If you suspect that your conditioner might be causing problems, there are several things you can do. 1) Use less of it next time. If your hair is short, use half the amount specified on the package. 2) Use conditioner only where you need it—on the ends of your hair, for example. 3) Dilute instant conditioner with water if you think it's too heavy for your hair. 4) Always rinse your hair twice as long as you normally would to remove all traces of conditioner.

 ## MASSAGE FOR HEALTHY HAIR

To give your conditioning program more clout, supplement it with a weekly scalp massage. This stimulates blood circulation to the hair follicles in the scalp, and is especially good for dry hair because it spreads oils. You can massage your scalp before shampooing or anytime you have a few moments to spare. One of the pluses of massage is that it's also a great way to relieve tension.

How to: Spread your fingers about an inch apart and place your fingertips on your scalp. Starting at the back or the front, knead your scalp gently all over, lifting your hair as you go. You should feel your scalp moving slightly beneath your fingertips. Massage all around the hairline at the front and sides of the head and at the nape of the neck. Never use your nails or massage vigorously, or you may damage your scalp or hair.

Another trick to rev up your scalp's circulation: Do a modified headstand. Kneel down on the floor with your forearms stretched out on the floor about a foot apart. Now lock your fingers together and place them palms up on the floor. Place the crown of your head between your hands and hold this position for a few minutes.

You can also get the blood flowing to your scalp by lying down on your back on the bed and letting your head dangle over the edge for a few moments.

2

GETTING THE THE RIGHT CUT

A pretty hairstyle can do wonders for your looks and give your spirits a boost. The secret behind a super hairstyle: a great cut that complements your face shape and suits your hair type. What goes into a good haircut? The following checklist will tell you.

- It should be easy to maintain and look almost as good when you style it as it did the day you walked out of the salon.
- It should hold its basic shape even in the worst weather.
- It should be versatile enough to offer more than one styling option, even if it's short.

If the haircut you have right now doesn't meet these guidelines, or if you have to fuss too much to get it into shape, it could be because it's all wrong for you. The fact is, certain haircuts work better than others for some types of hair, and some haircuts may not work at all for you.

There's no such thing as bad hair, but there are plenty of bad haircuts. Whether your hair is baby fine or coarse and bushy, it can look terrific with the right cut. So whatever you do, don't fight your natural hair type—go with it, and eventually you'll learn to love it.

THE PERFECT CUT FOR YOUR HAIR

The perfect cut takes advantage of your hair texture (fine, medium, or coarse) and degree of curl (straight, wavy, or curly). Chances are, you probably already know what type of hair you have, but just in case you don't here's a fast way to find out: Wash your hair, comb it out, and let it dry naturally. Fine hair takes about fifteen to twenty minutes to dry at the most; medium hair, twenty-five to thirty minutes; and coarse hair, forty-five minutes or longer. One look in the mirror after it's dry will tell you the degree of natural wave your hair has. Does it look stick-straight, slightly wavy, very wavy, or curly? In its natural state, curly fine hair tends to look frizzy instead of curly, and coarse curly hair can take on a wild, bushy appearance.

Now that you know what type of hair you have, you can get a cut that makes the most of it. Keep in mind that short hair is the easiest to maintain but the most limited in styling options. Long hair is the most versatile because you can wear it up or down, but upkeep can be time-consuming.

The best haircuts are hassle-free. They're neat and uncomplicated, but not severe—swingy hair is what to aim for. You can use accessories or styling tricks to add more dash to a basic cut. Here are the haircuts that go with, not against, your hair type.

- FINE HAIR A blunt cut will give you maximum fullness. It can fall anywhere from chin-length to shoulder-length. Any longer than that and it will look droopy—the weight of the hair will straighten out any natural wave or curl you have. To add interest, try bangs—straight, wispy, or brushed to one side. A very short, layered cut is excellent for straight fine hair, but avoid longish layers—they'll make your hair look choppy. Fine, slightly wavy hair looks pretty tapered at the sides for softness, perhaps with a sweep of bangs. Curly fine hair looks super in a short layered cut that frames the face. If your hair is very straight and baby fine, blowdry it for a sleek look. If you don't like bangs, consider a side part—it can change your whole look. You might also consider a body wave or a perm to give your hair more bulk. Setting lotions are another excellent way to add body to fine hair.

- MEDIUM-BODIED HAIR Lucky you. With this kind of hair, there are many styling options available to you. You can wear your hair short, shoulder length, or longer. If it's straight, a blunt cut will play up your hair's natural body. An angled style that's shorter at the sides and longer in back is a nice variation. A soft sweep of bangs brushed to one side works well on your hair, too. For added fullness, a slightly layered cut can be the answer. A short layered cut is the best way to enhance natural curls. For extra wave, set your hair on hot rollers or use a curling iron.

- COARSE HAIR With the wrong cut your type of hair can look bushy, especially if it's thick. Avoid extremes—very short styles that will make your hair stick out all over, or superlong ones that make your hair look wild. A style that's chin length or shoulder length with interest at the sides and front will help control it. If your hair is curly, avoid a blunt cut—it goes against your natural hair texture. There's no way it will look sleek and straight unless you blow it dry every day, which can be damaging to your hair. Try a short to medium-length, layered cut instead. Face-framing curls, for instance, will look fabulous on you. If you let your hair dry naturally it will look springier. If you set your hair, set it dry, on electric rollers, and leave them in for only a short time or you'll wind up with masses of uncontrollable curls.

Your hairstyle should agree with your skin type, too. If your skin breaks out where it comes in contact with your hair, such as underneath your bangs, switch to a different style. Meanwhile, try to keep your hair off that part of your face, and keep your skin sparkling clean.

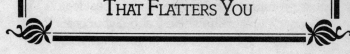

FIND THE STYLE THAT FLATTERS YOU

The shape of your face and your features have a lot to do with how attractive a given style will look on you. There's no such thing as a perfectly contoured face. It's true that almost any style works on an oval-shaped face, but if you don't have one, don't worry—many models don't either. The trick is to find a style that looks terrific on *you*, that's cut to suit *your* unique features.

The right style can play up your best features, help minimize your flaws. To get an idea of what style will look best on you, start by figuring out your face shape. To do this, wash your hair, then comb it back off your face. Now stand in front of a mirror and lightly trace the contour of your face on the mirror with a piece of soap. (Don't worry about getting the mirror dirty—a squirt of glass cleaner will take it right off.) Analyze the pattern you've just made. If it's widest at the forehead and cheeks and narrow at the chin, you have a heart-shaped face. Is it broadest at the forehead and jawline? Then your face shape is square. A diamond-shaped face is fullest at the center. A face that's narrow at the top and wide at the bottom is triangle shaped. If your face looks circular and you have full cheeks, its shape is round. A high forehead and square jaw usually mean a long angular face.

Next analyze your features. Study them head on and in profile. And be honest! Remember, nobody's perfect. Do you have a high or a low forehead? Is your nose prominent? Are your eyes your best feature? Is your neck long or short? How about your chin? Does it jut out, or does it recede? Do your ears stick out or lie flat?

If your hair is still wet, dry it as usual, then play with it a little. Tie it back or sweep it up. Pull a swatch of it over your forehead to see how you'd look with bangs. Comb your hair a different way. If you usually part it in the center, try a side part. Comb it forward if you usually wear it off your face. If it's long, hike it up a few inches to get an idea of how it would look shorter. Make a mental note of the effects you like best.

Finally, take a long look in a full-length mirror and review your build. It's important to take your overall proportions into account when choosing a hairstyle. Are you tall or short, slender or overweight?

Now it's time to put your research to work. Following are some of the most common face shapes and body types and the styles that flatter them, plus tips to help you camouflage your flaws. These aren't hard-and-fast rules because everyone's face shape is unique, but they will give you some general guidelines on how to wear your hair.

Face Shapes

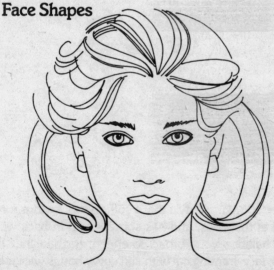

• ROUND The trick here is to make your face look thinner, more angular. A style with height at the crown and sides that curve around the chin will make your face look longer, trimmer. Soft waves starting at eye level will create angles. Graduated layers will add contours, play up your cheekbones. In a graduated style, the layers are not cut all over the head. They're shaped around the face, beginning at the bangs and becoming progressively longer toward the chin or shoulders—wherever the style ends. Don't part your hair in the center, pull it straight back off your face, or cut it supershort; your face will just look rounder. Another no: Styles that are fullest at cheek level.

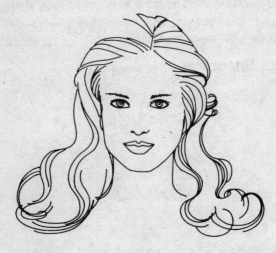

- **SQUARE** A style that's soft on top, swings forward at the sides, and has some length in back will help balance your broad forehead and jawline. A sleek, face-framing cut with soft curvy bangs will look great on you. Feathery curls at the sides, aiming toward or away from the face, will soften your features. Avoid styles that are flat on top.

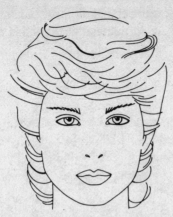

● TRIANGLE A style that gives you height and width at the crown and temples will help balance your broad chin. A curly style, cut above the jawline, would be especially pretty. Avoid styles that hit at cheekbone level.

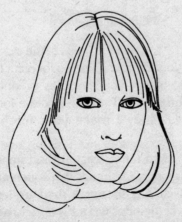

● DIAMOND To camouflage a narrow forehead and jawline, choose a style that falls softly from the temples to below the chin. Full curvy bangs will fill out the forehead. Avoid fullness at the sides and styles that are shorter than chin length.

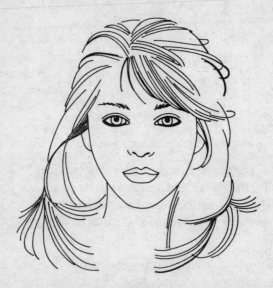

- HEART You need fullness at the sides to compensate for your narrow chin. Go for a cut that is layered starting below your temples or one with an off-center part and fluffy sides. Avoid a full fringe of heavy bangs—they'll make your forehead look broader.

- LONG Aim for interest at the forehead. Tendrils, curls or long wide bangs will soften angles and make your face look shorter. A medium-length style with fullness at the sides will add width to a long face. If your hair is long, a tousled mane of soft curls would be sensational. Avoid an angled cut that's shorter at the sides than in the back, or hair that hovers at chin length. If you pull your hair back off your face, let some tendrils escape to frame your face.

Facial Features

• HIGH FOREHEAD Bangs are ideal. Make them curly or feathery or brush them to one side. Gentle waves at the sides near the temples will also downplay a high broad forehead. You can wear your hair long or short, layered or straight, but avoid volume at the crown.

• LOW FOREHEAD A layered cut with fullness at the temples is a great style for you. A short fringe of soft bangs will make your forehead look longer. Another trick to fool the eye: Wear your hair back away from the face to make your forehead seem higher. You can wear your hair any length you like—but avoid parting it in the middle.

• PROMINENT NOSE What you may regard as your worst flaw could be your most distinctive feature—think of Barbra Streisand. Soft layers, wisps, or curls surrounding the face will diminish your nose. Short bangs that stop right above your brows draw the eyes up, away from the nose. A style with lift and movement shifts the focus of attention from the center of the face. Try a short curly cut with volume at the crown. If your hair is medium length, go for an angled cut that's shorter in back, longer in front. In general, long hair softens a prominent nose—just keep your hair swingy. Don't wear your hair stick-straight or part it down the center. If you slick your hair back, pull out some wisps around the face.

- **LARGE EARS** The best way to deal with protruding ears is to cover them up—any wavy or curly style will work. You can wear your hair short provided the tips of your ears are concealed. Avoid a blunt cut, especially if your hair is fine and straight, or your ears may peek through when your hair gets dirty. Consider a body wave or perm to add volume to your hair.

- **SHORT NECK** A layered style will make your neck look longer. Don't wear your hair long, straight, and all one length or your neck will seem to disappear beneath your locks.

- **LONG NECK** Width and fullness at the sides will make your neck look shorter. So will a medium-length blunt cut. Avoid extremely short styles that reveal a long stretch of neck.

- **RECEDING CHIN** Camouflage the flaw with a style that falls slightly below the jawline. Short full bangs add height at the crown and will draw attention away from your chin. Fullness at the chinline will also help.

- **PROMINENT JAW** Volume at the top of the head will help minimize a jaw that juts out too much. So will a below-chin-length cut, angled so it is long in back and shorter on the sides. Avoid full bangs.

- **PRETTY EYES** The old draw-the-eye trick is tried and true. If you call attention to a great feature, no one will notice your flaw. And bangs can make beautiful eyes the central attraction. Wear yours feathery, straight, spiked, short and fluffy—or long and full. The choice is up to you.

Body Types

- TALL AND THIN   A soft shoulder-length style is flattering and has an added bonus: It will camouflage narrow shoulders. Cascades of waves or curls offset an angular build. Avoid very short styles that can make your head look too small.

- SHORT AND PETITE   Your hairstyle should be in perfect proportion to your build. Good hairdressers will ask you to stand up before they begin cutting your hair, so they can judge what length will be most flattering. In general, you can go as short as you like. Close-cropped styles will look super on you. But beware of long hair or wild, way-out styles that can overpower you.

- OVERWEIGHT   If you're heavy, keep your hairstyle sleek and simple, chin to shoulder length. An overdone or busy look will emphasize your weight problem.

How to Get the Haircut You Want

There's nothing more exhilarating than getting a great haircut. But going to a salon can be intimidating. You may not know how to talk to a hairdresser or even how to go about finding a good one in the first place. Not knowing how much to tip can be traumatic too.

The first thing to do when contemplating a haircut, especially if you want to make a big change in your style, is to stop worrying about how things will turn out. All it takes is a little salon savvy to survive the experience and wind up loving your hair.

Tracking Down a Good Stylist

The best way to find a good hairdresser is to ask friends, relatives, even strangers whose hair you like, where they had theirs done. Don't go by a famous name alone. Just because a salon is well known doesn't mean it guarantees a good cut.

If you live in a small town, check with a large department store in your area to find out if it has a hair salon. Many reputable hair styling chains with well-trained stylists work out of major department stores.

After you've found a salon, you might want to drop in for a few minutes before you make an appointment. Remember, a little research can prevent a haircut you'll be unhappy with later. Don't feel uncomfortable about just observing. Try to time your visit during the salon's busiest hours so you'll get a better idea of what kind of work is being done there.

Don't be fooled by a glitzy decor. Look past the glamorous trappings and focus on the haircuts in progress. A very trendy salon that gives the latest, most sophisticated cuts may not be for you. On the other hand, a salon that seems stodgy or isn't up on the newest styles may be one to avoid also. Pay special attention to customers who have the same type of hair you do. Do the haircuts in progress fit the individual or does everyone come out looking the same? Do the hairstylists seem rushed, intent on moving customers in and out at lightning speed? Or is the pace relaxed and pleasant? If, overall, you get a good feeling about the salon and like most of the cuts you see, then you've found the right place. If you like only a few cuts or if the atmosphere seems frenzied, keep on looking.

Consider a Consultation

Once you've decided upon a salon, you might want to schedule a free consultation before you actually have your hair cut. A consultation is a good idea if you're considering a major change, such as a perm, or if you want to go from a long to a short style. It's also a golden opportunity to get acquainted with the hairdresser and build up rapport. Feel free to ask all the questions you want: How much will it cost? Can you maintain the look yourself? Even if you don't opt for a consultation, make it a point to find out fees before you schedule an appointment. All it takes is a quick phone call. In most salons, a standard cut includes a shampoo and blowdry. Sometimes, though, you can skip one or both of these steps and save yourself some money. But find out in advance what the salon's policy is.

Do Your Homework

Always have a fairly clear idea of what you want before you arrive at the salon. Flip through a few women's magazines and pick out some styles that appeal to you, then clip them out and take them along. They don't have to be exactly what you want. You might have one picture that shows the style you like, another that shows the amount of wave you want from a perm. Most hairdressers appreciate your input and the pictures can serve as a helpful starting point in discussing the best style for you. If your hairdresser doesn't think the styles you have in mind are right for your hair type or face shape, he or she will make suggestions. For instance, if the style you want works best on wavy hair and yours is straight, he or she might recommend a body wave or perm.

A good stylist should be attentive, pleasant, willing to answer your questions, and should make you feel secure about how you'll look after the job's done. If the hairstylist you see comes across as a prima donna or tries to foist his or her ideas on you, it's perfectly okay to get up and leave before the work starts. Better to suffer a few moments of embarrassment than to live for months with a style you don't like. In reality, most stylists aim to please and will take your suggestions seriously. Sometimes a hairdresser will make a suggestion that you may not be sure about— a body wave to add volume to fine hair, for example. Tell him or her you'll think about it, but for now, you're not ready to make such a big change. Usually, the style you end up with is a compromise between your ideal and what will work best with your hair type.

Be Realistic

It's important to be realistic about what a haircut can

and cannot accomplish. No haircut can make short hair longer, of course, but a perm will add volume. Neither will a new haircut make you more popular, turn you into a cover-girl beauty, take off weight, or add inches to your height.

Some girls cut their hair for all the wrong reasons. When not to have your hair cut: if you've just broken up with your boyfriend or found out that you didn't make the cheerleading team. You might be tempted to make a drastic change in your hair because you can't make real changes in your life. If you're down in the dumps, resist the urge to cut your hair until you're feeling better. Or consider making a minor change—having bangs cut if you don't already have them, or layering the sides of your hair.

Speak Up

Communicating with the stylist is the key to getting the cut you want. Hairdressers aren't mind readers; you have to tell them what you want. Let yours know how much time you want to spend maintaining your hair and how good you are at styling it. If you're all thumbs with a blowdrier, or if sports are a major part of your life, you need an easy-care hairstyle. If you don't mind spending a little more time fixing your hair, you can try a more elaborate look.

Also tell your stylist about what you've done to your hair within the past year—whether you've had it permed or straightened or used henna on it. If you've had any problems with your hair—split ends that keep coming back, or a perm that ruined your hair—tell your hairdresser, and ask for advice.

You should also let your stylist in on any recent health problems you've had; illness can affect the way your hair behaves.

Be Specific

Before your stylist starts snipping, make sure he or she knows how much you want cut off. Be specific. "An inch off all around and long bangs, about eyebrow level," doesn't leave much room for error. If your hair is layered and you want to let it grow out, say so, or you'll have to wait another month or two before you can begin. By the time the stylist takes scissors in hand, you should know exactly what's being done and have a pretty clear picture of what your hair will look like when the job's finished.

Watch closely as your hairdresser works, especially during the styling stage as it's being blown dry and combed or brushed into shape. Ask for tips on how to style your hair yourself, how often you should condition it, any tricks you can use to make your new style look different for everyday and special occasions.

If the worst occurs and your hairdresser cuts off too much, try to keep calm. Maybe there was a good reason for cutting off that extra inch—to get rid of split ends or to even out your hair. But if you asked for a trim and got a short cut, make it clear that you're dissatisfied. And in this case, you're definitely not obligated to leave a tip. It's possible you won't be charged at all if the stylist knows you're unhappy. If he or she didn't cut enough, ask if you can come back in a week for another trim. Most hairstylists will oblige without charging you. You wanted shorter bangs? This is no problem at all. The hairdresser can snip them shorter right then and there.

The standard tip is fifteen percent, plus a dollar or two for the stylist's assistant who shampooed your hair or rolled it on perm rods. Salon owners usually don't expect a tip at all.

 ## Living with a New Look

Normally, it takes a few days to adjust to the new you, longer if you've made a big change. You may find yourself taking sneak peeks in the mirror every so often and wondering if that's really you who's staring back. The bigger the change, the longer it will take you to get used to it. Keep in mind that any haircut looks best a few weeks later, after it's settled into its new shape. The sooner you start caring for your hair and styling it, the faster you'll adjust.

Coping with a Haircut You Hate

Before you say you hate your hair, live with it a while. You may wind up loving it after you've gotten used to the new look, and may even decide to have your hair cut the same way again. If you really don't like it after a few weeks, you don't have to wear scarves for the next few months.

Here are some options: If it's not too short, you can have it recut (by a different stylist) to give it a better line. Or consider a perm—curls can camouflage a multitude of sins. This is an especially good solution if your hair's been shorn—a perm gives short hair more volume. Or wait a few months until your hair is a workable length, then consult with a new hairdresser about a solution.

Other tricks you can try: Experiment with makeup, so your face becomes the focal point instead of your hair. Wear bright colors to give your spirits a lift and draw the eye away from your hair. Frilly clothes will make you feel more feminine; crazy accessories will also shift attention away from your hair. Chances are your hair doesn't look as bad as you think it does. The style probably just doesn't match the image you have of yourself.

How to Recognize a Great Cut

A good cut has swing and bounce and falls into place without much fussing. It should have a sleek line with no straggly ends or tufts that stick out. But the real test of a haircut is how well you like it. It should fit your personal style as well as your life-style. Another clue to a good cut: It should be easy to maintain. Any hairstyle that takes more than a half hour to fix is too complicated. If you get compliments on your hair and feel comfortable with it, the style probably reflects the real you, and that, after all, is what a great haircut is all about.

In general, it's best to leave haircutting to the pros, but if you have long straight hair that's all one length, there's no reason why you can't trim it yourself. Or better yet, have a friend trim it for you. It's more fun that way, and another pair of eyes will help ensure that it comes out even. You'll need a pair of sharp hair-cutting scissors four-and-a-half to six inches long (available at beauty supply stores), a wide-tooth comb, some large clips or bobby pins, a roll of hair-setting tape, a spritzing bottle, and a hand-held mirror for a clear view of the back of your head. Pick a well-lit spot to do the cutting. When deciding how much to cut, keep in mind that your hair will shrink about half an inch when it dries.

1. First, shampoo your hair and condition it. Then towel dry it and comb out the tangles. Next make a center part and comb your hair until it's smooth and straight. Wrap on a towel sarong-style so your shoulders are exposed—shirt collars can get in the way of cutting and block your view.

2. Begin at the sides. Separate the hair from the ear forward and twirl it into a giant curl; clip or pin it up out of the way.

3. Next, divide the hair in back horizontally into equal sections, pinning up all but the bottom section. Four or five sections is the norm, but if your hair is exceptionally thick you may need to make more sections.

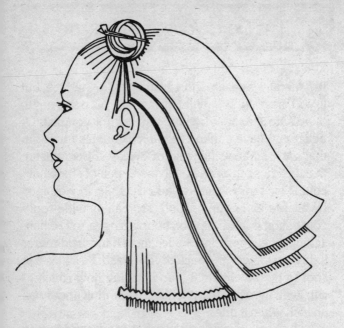

4. Comb out the bottom layer. Place a piece of hair-setting tape just above where you want to cut. Then slowly, smoothly cut straight across, making sure to hold your head still. Check to make sure that the ends are even before going on. Uncoil the next section and cut it the same length as the first one, using setting tape as a guideline. Continue in the same manner until you've cut all sections. Spray hair now and then to keep it wet during cutting.

    5. Now unpin either of the side sections. Divide it in half horizontally, then repin the top section. Comb the section you've just separated straight down in front of your ear. Never cut over your ear, or your hair

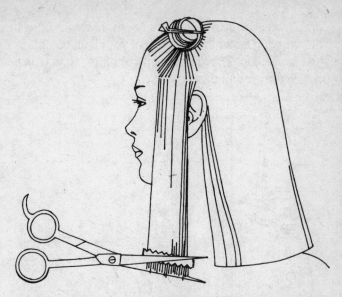

will come out uneven. Place a piece of hair-setting tape even with the back section and cut straight across. Now bring down the top layer, comb it out, and cut it the same length as the bottom layer. (If your hair is very thick, you might want to divide the side hair into more than two sections.) Repeat this procedure on the other side.

6. Comb out your hair, blending sides into back, and check for any straggly ends. That's all there is to it—you've just given yourself a professional cut. Blowdry and style as usual.

How to Cut Your Own Bangs

The secret behind beautiful fluffy bangs is frequent trimming. Messy bangs that dangle in your eyes aren't very attractive. It might seem that your bangs are growing faster than the rest of your hair, but this is just an illusion. They're right on your face, so you just notice the growth there more.

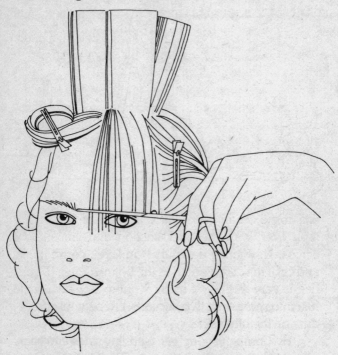

You can keep your bangs looking neat between haircuts by trimming them yourself, but there's a trick to it. If you've ever botched the job, it's probably because you pulled all the hair to the center of your forehead and snipped it straight across in one big clump. The problem with cutting your bangs this way is that the sides, near the temples, will come out longer. Or you might have cut off too much. Remember that your bangs will look shorter when they dry, so just cut off a quarter of an inch for the best results. It's better to have your bangs a little long than much too short. Follow these instructions and you can't go wrong.

1. Pull back all your hair except the bangs and wet them with a mister. Now slick your bangs off your face.

2. Comb down a thin horizontal section (about a third of the bangs) and pin the rest back. Comb the section straight down. Now divide it in half. Holding your hair between your index and middle fingers, snip straight across, slowly—don't rush. Repeat the same procedure for the other half.

3. Comb down half of the remaining bangs and blend into the hair you've just cut. Divide your bangs in half again. Trim one half at a time to the same length as the first layer.

4. Bring down the last section and cut it the same way.

Tip: You don't have to shampoo all of your hair if only your bangs are dirty. To wash your bangs, wet them thoroughly, then apply a little bit of shampoo and rub it into your bangs. Work up a lather, then rinse. Towel dry and comb.

3

POINTERS
ON
PERMS

If you're longing for cascades of waves or luxurious curls, or if you just want to give your hair a body boost, a perm could be the answer. Perms have come a long way since the crimped styles of Grandma's day. Then perming was a time-consuming and unpleasant process involving strong solutions and curlers that hooked up to a heat machine. Not anymore. Today's perms are safe, gentle, and more natural-looking than ever. And they won't hurt your hair one bit if done properly.

PERK UP YOUR HAIR WITH A PERM

A perm can give fine limp hair body and fullness, make thin hair look more abundant, and turn straight hair into a tumble of soft waves or curls. If you have fine frizzy hair, a perm can bend those frizzies into curls. The way your hair looks after a perm depends on its texture and length, the type of rollers used, the strength of the perm solution, and how long it's left on your hair.

There are two main types of perms. If you want to add body and volume to your hair, a body wave is what you need. To wave or curl your hair, you'll want a real permanent. It's called a "permanent" for a good reason. The chemicals in a permanent wave solution penetrate to the heart of the hairshaft and break down its structure so your hair will take on a new shape.

Here's how it's done:

First waving solution is applied to soften the hair and make it accept the shape of the rods it's wrapped on. The degree of curl is determined by the size of the

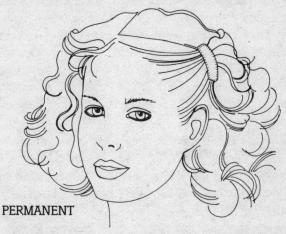

PERMANENT

rods used. After about ten to twenty minutes of processing time, the waving solution is rinsed out and a neutralizer is applied which stops the curling action and fixes the curl into shape. Then the neutralizer is washed out and your permanent is finished.

Consider carefully before you opt for a perm. It's a look you'll have to live with. There's no way to get rid of a perm once you have one without putting more chemicals on your hair or cutting off the permed portion as your hair grows out. If you're having your perm done in a salon, discuss with your hairdresser the kind of look you want. Pull out that picture you've been saving and show your stylist exactly what you have in mind. If you want a style that you can just wash and dry naturally, you should probably go the wavy or curly route. A body wave won't change the

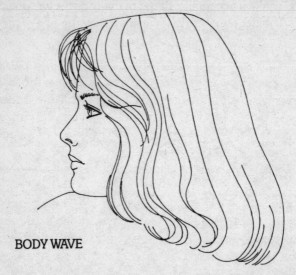

BODY WAVE

natural texture of your hair dramatically—it mainly acts as a body booster and imparts a slight degree of wave so you can still blowdry and style your hair as usual.

Have It Done Your Way

Perms can be given in several different ways depending on the look you want to create. To add volume you can have the underlayer of your hair permed and leave the top layer untouched. For more lift, you can have your hair permed close to the roots. If your hair is curlier in some spots than others, you can have a partial perm to make the irregular parts blend in with the rest.

Preperm Prep

Always have your hair cut before a perm. Otherwise you may have to snip off some of your new curls later on. A perm has more body and fullness when done on hair that's cut in layers.

Long straight hair is the most difficult to perm. The waving solution might not penetrate the hair evenly when it's wound on rollers, and the added weight of long hair tends to straighten out the curl. In addition, the hair may look straight at the roots and wavy on the ends as it grows out.

It's a good idea to give your hair a deep conditioning treatment before you perm it to get it in tip-top shape. Don't perm your hair at all if it's dry or broken, or if it's been exposed to any other chemical process such as bleaching. If you're in doubt about whether or not your hair can stand up to a perm, have a test curl done.

Home Perming

If you're giving yourself a home perm, follow the package instructions to the letter. Never assume that one brand can be used the same way as another, and be careful to choose a perm kit that produces the type of curl you want. The package label will tell you what kind of results to expect. "Body only," "soft body," "regular," and "extracurly" are some of the descriptions you'll come across.

Perm Pampering

Wait at least forty-eight hours after a perm before you shampoo your hair—washing it too soon can relax the curl before it's had time to set. Your hair might have a faint chemical odor after a perm, but that will go away after a few shampoos. In the meantime, you can spray your hair with cologne to keep it sweet-smelling. Another side effect of perming: Your hair might turn a little lighter in color.

Permed hair requires kid-glove treatment because the chemicals you put on it make it more fragile. There are products made especially for use on permed hair that you can buy through salons. In any case, use a mild shampoo and follow up with an instant conditioner. A deep-conditioning treatment every three to four weeks is a must. Use a wide-tooth comb to remove snarls. Bend over and comb your hair gently from nape to crown to prevent unnecessary pulling on the hair. Easy does it with brushing too. Excess heat will damage permed hair, so if you blowdry it use the warm or cool setting.

A curly perm will look best if you let it dry naturally, then fluff it up with a comb or brush. You can perk up your perm in the morning or anytime your hair has fallen flat; just mist it with water and your curls will come back to life. If your perm begins to look droopy, it's probably time for a trim. This will help revive the curls.

The average perm lasts about four months, depending on the type of solution used and the natural texture of your hair. It will usually grow out faster on fine hair than on coarse hair, but before you have another perm make sure that all of the old one is out, and that your hair is in good condition. A body wave has an even shorter life-span because it's produced with a milder solution.

The Best Time to Perm

There's no perfect time to perm your hair, but be aware that summer sun, salt water, and chlorine—which can dry out even unprocessed hair—can damage permed hair. Frequent washing and working with the hair, which you're more likely to do in warm weather, tend to relax the curl, too. And summer humidity can turn a perm into frizz fast.

If you're planning to spend a lot of time at the seashore, cover up your hair with a hat or scarf to protect it from the damaging ultraviolet rays of the sun. And while you're basking on the beach, apply a deep conditioner with a wide-tooth comb and slick your hair back. The heat of the sun will make it penetrate more effectively. The conditioner will also protect your hair from the drying effects of salt water.

Experiment with Styles

The wonderful thing about a body wave or perm is the freedom it gives you. You won't have to set it or spend hours rolling it anymore. And it opens up a whole new world of styling options that never worked when your hair lacked body or curl.

Consider wearing some hair accessories, for instance. Pull your hair back off your face by anchoring it with some combs at the sides—they'll stay in now. A ribbon or bandanna looks great tied on full bouncy hair. A pair of colorful barrettes will peek prettily out of the waves in permed hair. If your hair is longish, pull it back with a barrette, fluff up your bangs if you have them, and leave a few wisps free at the sides for a soft romantic look. There's no end to the looks you can create.

Perm Problems Solved

If your perm turns out to be a disaster—either it didn't take or it looks like one big ball of frizz—don't panic. It might not be as bad as you think. You have to understand what went wrong before you can take steps to make it right. If your perm didn't take, it might be because the waving solution was rinsed off too soon or because the neutralizing solution that locks in the curl wasn't left on long enough. You can have your perm redone. How soon depends upon the condition of your hair. A good hairdresser can advise you.

If your hair turned out too curly or frizzy, there is a way to reverse the process, but it should only be done in the salon. The same chemicals that were used to wave the hair are combed through to loosen the curl. All these chemicals can be hard on the hair. Before attempting to reverse your perm, make sure your hair is strong enough to stand more processing.

Hair that's dull and dry after a perm is a sign of overprocessing—the waving solution was left on too long. Use a hot oil treatment once or twice a week until the condition of your hair improves.

How to Live with a Perm You Hate

If you really hate your perm, there are many ways to make it look better until it grows out. Using a creme rinse after every shampoo will help relax the curl. Conditioning on a regular basis will tame frizzies and help restore luster to damaged hair. You can have your hair shaped or cut shorter to remove some of the curl. Try blowdrying your hair to give it a smoother look—but don't do it every day, or you'll dry it out. Headbands, barrettes, and other hair accessories will help keep very curly or bushy locks off your face and under control. The main thing to remember, though, is that any perm relaxes over time.

 ## GETTING IT STRAIGHT

If you were blessed with curly hair, think twice before you decide to have it straightened. Many girls with straight hair would love to have your curly locks. It's true that curly hair can be hard to handle, but straightening isn't the only way to keep it under control. Maybe you just need a good cut that complements your hair texture. Hair straightening is one of the harshest things you can do to your hair. However, if you're convinced that only straight hair will make you happy, proceed—with caution. The chemicals used in hair straighteners are similar to those in depilatories; they can break your hair or actually dissolve it if they're too strong or left on too long.

The Hazards of Hair Straightening

A hair straightener is like a perm in reverse. A chemical solution is combed through the hair to soften it and relax the curl, then rinsed out. After that, a neutralizer is applied to hold the hair in its new shape. One of the reasons straightening is so hazardous is because it's applied close to the scalp—which can result in irritation. Perms are less likely to irritate the scalp because most of the waving solution ends up on the hair that's wound around the perm rods instead.

No straightener can make your hair perfectly straight without doing quite a bit of damage at the same time. The kinkiest type of hair is finer and harder to straighten than coarse hair because it's more fragile. And the best a straightener can do is relax very curly or kinky hair. Never straighten your hair if it's dry or brittle, or if it's dyed or bleached. If your scalp is flaky, scratched, or sensitive in any way, wait until the condition clears up before straightening your hair.

Play It Safe

The safest way to have your hair straightened is in the salon by a good hairdresser who's an expert at it. Remember, this is serious business. A professional will have the know-how to use the straightener correctly and leave it on for the right length of time to achieve the results you want. Always tell the hairdresser how straight you want your hair to be. And prepare your hair for processing by giving it a deep conditioning treatment beforehand.

As your hair grows out, have only the portion close to the scalp restraightened. Repeating the whole process can cause breakage or make your hair overly dry or brittle. You can safely straighten your hair about twice a year, unless a reputable hairdresser gives you the go-ahead to do it more often.

If you decide to take on the project at home, always follow instructions on home straightening kits to the letter. Do a strand test to check how your hair will turn out. Before you apply the neutralizer, make sure your hair is free of tangles—this is the step that fixes your hair in its new shape. Don't attempt home straightening at all if your hair is extremely curly or kinky—only a professional can successfully work with this type of hair.

Be Kind to Straightened Hair

Straightened hair is fragile and deserves all the pampering you can give it. Use a mild shampoo and an instant conditioner. Comb and brush as gently as possible. Give your hair a hot oil treatment every three to four weeks to restore gloss and moisture. Cut down on the use of curling irons and hot curlers—more than twice a week is too much. Blowdry your hair on the warm or cool setting. Protect your hair with a bathing cap when you go swimming, and keep your head covered at the beach and during outdoor activities when it's likely to become snarled.

If you're unhappy about how your hair turned out after straightening, don't redo it. Give your hair a chance to rest. Then go to a salon and check with an expert to find out when you can safely try it again.

Be aware that repeated straightenings will damage your hair, especially if it's long. If your hair is dry and brittle, step up conditioning by giving your hair a hot oil treatment once or twice a week. Split or broken ends are also common signs of trouble. Have your hair trimmed to remove the damaged portion, and lavish conditioner on parched ends.

4

STYLING
SAVVY

Styling tools and a little know-how are all you need to do your hair like a pro. There's a wide variety of equipment available ranging from blowdriers to hot rollers to curling wands. With practice and a few pointers, they're simple to use. You can't *create* a style with these tools; they're designed as aids to help you maintain your hair, touch it up, make it look special. If you don't have a good haircut to begin with, even the best equipment won't help. Here's how to put these gadgets to work for you.

ALL ABOUT BLOWDRYING

Your hairdresser blowdries your hair in a flash with a few flourishes and flicks of the wrist. It looks so easy, but when you get home and try it yourself you're all thumbs. . . . Blowdrying looks easy because it is easy. Your hairdresser has the technique down pat. And you can master it too. The first thing to do is show your blowdrier who's boss. Take charge of it; it's only a tool.

The best blowdrier for home styling is one that's not too powerful. A thousand watts or less is sufficient. The blowdrier should be lightweight, easy to grip, with two or more heat settings. Some come with attachments that fit onto the nozzle. One that's especially useful is a diffuser, which looks something like a large shower head. The purpose of the diffuser is to regulate the flow of air so that it spreads more evenly, instead of coming out in one big blast.

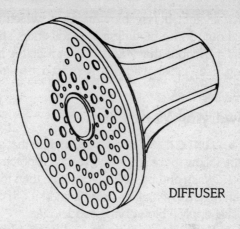

DIFFUSER

Unbreakable Blowdrying Rules

It's a fact: Heat isn't good for your hair. Overblowdrying can sap your hair of oils so that it looks dry and dull and breaks easily. When done correctly and with moderation, blowdrying won't damage your hair. Here are some rules to follow to prevent blowdrying abuse.

Always blowdry your hair on the warm or cool setting. And keep your blowdrier in constant motion. Aiming at one spot for any length of time can damage your hair. For the same reason, you should hold your blowdrier at least six to eight inches from your hair. Try not to use a blowdrier every day—your hair can only take so much heat before it shows signs of damage.

The most common mistake is to dry the hair until it's bone dry. Blowdry your hair so that it's still a little damp when you're finished. To protect your hair from heat, there are special conditioners made to apply to your hair right before blowdrying it, which are not rinsed out. Some blowdrying conditioners spray on; others are lotions that you comb through the hair. For styling, use a brush with widely spaced, heat-resistant plastic bristles.

Blowdrying Made Easy

• BLUNT CUTS   For blowdrying hair that's all one length, follow these steps and you can't botch the job.

1. Wash and condition your hair, then towel dry it. Gently remove tangles using a wide-tooth comb. If you like, apply a blowdrying conditioner.

2. Bend from the waist and begin blowdrying your hair at the nape of neck, gently combing through it with your fingers. Rotate the blowdrier to the sides and then up to the crown until your hair is about three-quarters dry. Then straighten up, flip your hair back in place, and comb or brush out snarls.

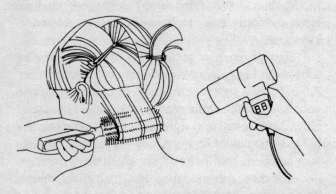

3. To style, start at the back and dry hair by sections from nape to crown, clipping up the rest of your hair to keep it out of your way. Scoop a section of hair no more than two inches thick onto your brush and roll it under twice to make sure it's secure. (Taking too much hair on your brush is a common mistake.) Now turn on the blower for a few seconds, and dry the rolled section of hair from ends to roots. Leave the hair curled around the brush for a second or two to set it, then gently unwind. Continue sectioning and drying the hair all the way up to the crown.

4. Now move on to the sides. Start with the bottom layer and roll and dry the same way as in the back, clipping up the rest of your hair to keep it from mixing with the section you're drying.

5. Finish by lightly running a brush through your hair. You may notice a few wiry ends sticking up at the crown that mar an otherwise beautiful blowdrying job. To smooth them down, pour a tiny bit of setting lotion onto your palm and run your hand over your hair. Setting lotion adds body to the hair and helps it hold a set. It comes in liquid or gel form. There are setting lotions for all hair types. Liquid setting lotions are the best because they're lightweight. Gels can make the hair sticky or gummy.

• LAYERED HAIR   To blowdry layered hair, try this technique: Shampoo and condition your hair, towel dry it, and comb it into place. Then, starting in the back, brush your hair in the opposite direction from how you want it to go while blowing it dry, to give the hair lift. Do the same thing on the sides, then in front. When your hair is almost dry, brush it the way you want it to go. To turn under straggly ends, roll a section of hair around the brush, and switch on the blower for a few seconds, using first the warm, then the cool setting.

- CURLS The best way to dry curly or permed hair is with a blowdrier made especially for your hair type or with one that has a diffuser attachment. These styling aids won't flatten out your curls the way a regular blowdrier will. When your hair is almost dry, shape it into place with your fingers.

- BANGS For full fluffy bangs, roll hair under and around the brush. Direct a stream of air on bangs for a few seconds, then gently unroll the brush.

Feathery bangs are done a different way. Pick up a section of hair on your brush and roll back and away from the face. Move the drier back and forth across the bangs, then remove the brush.

 # HANDLING HOT ROLLERS

Hot rollers produce a looser curl than regular rollers, but they come in handy when you want to add body and fullness to your hair or create waves or curls quickly. Hot rollers come as a unit. They are heated on pegs that are attached to an electric plate. You plug the unit into the wall and when the rollers reach the right temperature, you take them off the pegs and roll your hair around them as you would on regular curlers. Look for a unit made by a reputable manufacturer. It will be thermostatically controlled, which means that the curlers will stop heating automatically when they reach the proper temperature. Never use a model that isn't thermostatically controlled—it can overheat and damage your hair.

There are several different types of hot roller units available—regular, water-misting, and conditioning mist models. The regular and water-misting units are fine for all types of hair. The only difference between the two is that the gentle mist produced by the water-misting model lubricates the hair and makes it easier to roll up. The conditioning mist type is best for hair that's naturally dry or that has been damaged from perming, coloring, or other abuse. A conditioner, which protects the hair from heat, comes out in the mist.

Hot-roller kits come with large- medium- and small-sized rollers. The larger the roller you use, the softer the curl will be. Here are some tips to help you get great results when using hot rollers.

• Never set your hair when it's wet. Leave hot rollers in your hair for only a short time—about five to fifteen minutes. They're not designed to dry the hair. If you set your hair wet, the curl won't take at all. Blowdry your hair first or let it air dry naturally until just damp. To give the set more holding power, mist your hair lightly with setting lotion.

• Comb out all tangles before you put the rollers in your hair.

• To keep the ends of your hair from drying out from the heat and to prevent ridges, use end papers to roll up your hair. How to: Separate a section of hair and sandwich the ends between the fold in the end paper, then roll the hair around the curler. Squares of toilet paper, folded in half, can be used as end papers.

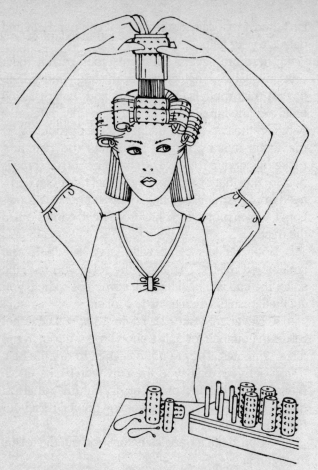

● Wind rollers carefully to prevent tangling. Don't wrap too much hair around them, or your set won't hold. Always use the fasteners that come with the kit to secure rollers—bobby pins and clips aren't strong enough to keep them in place. If you lose some fasteners, you can pick up more at a beauty supply store.

- For maximum curl, keep the rollers in until they've cooled off completely. If you just want to add body or a little wave, take them out sooner.
- Remove rollers carefully, working up from nape to crown to prevent tangles. If some of your hair becomes snarled, work the roller out gently without tugging.
- Don't brush your hair immediately. Wait a few moments for your hair to cool off. Then brush lightly to avoid flattening out the curls.
- Don't use hot rollers every day—the heat will damage and dry out your hair. At most, use them three times a week.

 ## CURLING WAND TIPS

This little gadget is terrific for perking up hair that's fallen flat, or for creating curls, waves, and tendrils. The beauty of a curling wand is that you can control exactly where you want to put a curl—all it takes is a flick of the wrist. A Teflon-coated curling wand with steaming unit will be the kindest to your hair, and lessen the chance of drying it out. It should be thermostatically controlled so you won't burn your hair.

How to: Make sure the wand is filled with water. Your hair should be clean and dry. Now slip a section of hair under the clip, making sure the ends are clamped inside it to prevent ridges. Roll the hair around the wand in the same direction you would if you were setting it on rollers—stopping short of the

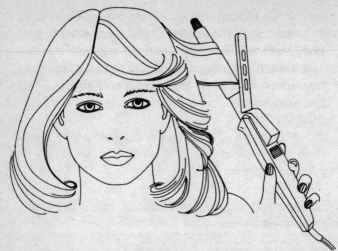

scalp. Always keep the heated wand clear of the scalp to prevent burning yourself. When you've rolled up the curl, press the steaming button briefly and hold the wand in place for about ten seconds. You can use two hands to grip the handle if it's easier that way. Unwind the hair, then go on to the next curl. Don't use a curling wand every day—it can damage your hair.

MORE STYLING AND SETTING TRICKS

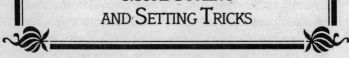

No matter what kind of hair you have—short or long, wavy or straight—there are all kinds of ways to make it look sensational without using any gadgets at all. You can make waves, add body, create curls or straighten them out with a few easy tricks. You can do some of them with material you have around the house such as tissue paper, pencils, or pipe cleaners. For others, all you need is a brush, and for the simplest ones, you can let your fingers do styling. The tricks that follow are all fast and fun.

Pin Curls

Your grandmother used them for a good reason—they work! They create lots of waves or bouncy curls, depending on how you use them. You can place just a few around your face or set all of your hair. For bouncy curls, apply a setting lotion first.

How to: Comb out a strand of hair and wind it around your finger. Fasten with a clip or bobby pin that has a coated tip. Don't use rusty clips or uncoated bobby pins—they can scratch the scalp. When your hair is dry, brush it out gently. Try pulling it back with a ribbon for a pretty effect.

Finger Fluffing

To add volume to wavy or curly hair that's short to medium length, this trick is tops and it's incredibly easy to do. Here's how: Shampoo your hair and towel dry it. Begin anywhere, and gently run your fingers through your hair as if you were combing it, lifting it up and out at the same time. Continue lifting and fluffing until your hair is nearly dry. Then comb or brush it lightly into shape. A fine misting of setting lotion applied when your hair is wet will give your hair even more body.

Another option: Let your hair dry naturally—don't use a blowdrier or you'll spoil the effect. Then, when your hair is completely dry, run your fingers through it to ruffle up the curls. For softer curls, lightly lift the hair with a "pick" (a comb that has about ten widely spaced prongs, instead of teeth) or with a styling brush. For a fabulous finish, put on a snappy headband or clip on a couple of barrettes.

Hair Wrapping

Hair wrapping is a safe and simple way to straighten out long hair that's wavy, curly, or frizzy. For it to work, your hair has to be soaking wet. First wet your hair,

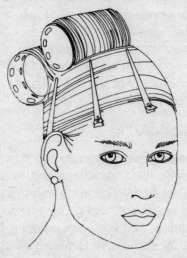

comb it out, and apply a setting lotion. Then set the hair at the crown on one or two big rollers. Now, starting at the temple, wrap your hair across your forehead and around the back of your head, smoothing it down as you go. Use large clips to secure the hair ends. Don't wrap your hair so tightly that you pull it, but be sure to keep the ends smooth. When your hair is dry, remove the clips and brush out. If your hair isn't perfectly straight, dampen it slightly with a mister and wrap it in the opposite direction.

Braiding

For tons of tiny waves, nothing beats braiding as a way of setting your hair. Even if you have the kind of hair that's stick straight, this trick will make it look full and fluffy. Braiding is done easiest with hair that's all one length.

For a very crimped look, dampen your hair first and braid it wet. Starting on one side of your part, make skinny braids and secure them with tiny elastic bands. (Small ones won't hurt your hair if you're careful with them.) Next braid the other side of your hair, then the crown and back. If you don't want to take the time to make real braids, you can take a shortcut by twisting two strands of hair together instead of the usual three. Your braids don't have to be lined up in regular rows, but they should be neatly twisted to prevent the rubber bands from tearing your hair when you remove them.

Leave the braids in until your hair dries, or as long as you like. But the longer you leave them in, the tighter the waves will be. Braid all of your hair or just some of it. You can even braid some sections halfway to create a different look. When you're ready to un-braid, remove the bands gently. If one gets stuck in your hair, snip it out with a small pair of scissors, being careful not to cut away any hair with it. Now brush out your hair. You'll be amazed at how full it looks.

Twisting

If you have medium-length to long hair, you'll love this trick. It will give your hair more body and create soft, loose waves—and it's a cinch to do. You can set your hair damp or dry depending on how much wave you want.

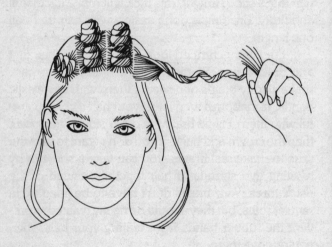

Here's how to do it: Starting anywhere, take a thin section of hair and twist it until it looks like a long corkscrew. Form the hair into a coil and secure it with a small hairpin. Continue to twist and coil all of your hair. After it dries, unwind the coils and comb out, using your fingers to fluff out your hair even more.

Pipe Cleaners

Pipe cleaners are a great alternative to rollers, and you probably have some around the house. You can use them on any length hair. The effect you'll get: lots of full loose waves. Dampen your hair and spray it with setting lotion first for more body. Then bend the pipe cleaners into a "U" shape. If your hair is thick, twist two pipe cleaners together to form a sturdier curler. Starting at the crown, comb out a thin section of hair and roll it up and around the pipe cleaner, then twist the pipe cleaner ends together to close. Now move on to the sides and back until all of your hair is set. Let your hair air dry, then take out the pipe cleaners and brush out. Don't overbrush, or you'll take out some of the curl.

Chopsticks

If you have straight hair that's all one length, you'll want to try this trick. It's perfect for fine, medium-length hair. The result you'll get: rows of softly rippling waves. First, dampen your hair, spray it with setting lotion and part it as you usually do. Starting on one side of the part, separate a section of hair horizontally. Comb it out and wind it under and around the stick. Secure underneath with a bobby pin. Continue down the side forming neat horizontal rows. Then move on to the other side and the back, using one stick per row. Let your hair dry naturally, then brush out.

Tissue Paper or Saran Wrap

For short or long hair, if you want to create gentle waves and add fullness, this set will do the job. First cut out six-inch strips of tissue paper or Saran Wrap and twist each one in the center. Spray your hair with setting lotion and comb out a strand. Place the strand of hair in the center of a strip and roll it up to the scalp, then tie. Repeat the process for each strand, wait about half an hour to forty-five minutes, then unroll your hair and softly brush.

Brush Set

Anytime your hair needs a quick lift, a round, wide-bristle plastic styling brush can come to the rescue. If your hair is cut in layers around your face, you can use a brush to form waves. Just scoop up a section of hair onto the brush and roll it back, away from the face. Be sure to wind it loosely to prevent the brush from becoming tangled in your hair. Leave the brush in for about ten minutes, then gently unwind. If your bangs look deflated, the brush trick can put the bounce back into them. Or you can turn under the ends of your hair. Roll ends under and around a brush and leave it in place for a few minutes before unwinding. For short hair, use a smaller brush.

Soft Rollers

The newest kind of rollers are soft and flexible. They're great for making bouncy curls and are much simpler to use than the metal, plastic, or mesh kind. That's because you don't have to roll them in neat rows or put them in with bobby pins. Plus, they're gentler on your hair than the rigid kind. Some are made of sponge; others are covered with fabric and look like large string beans. They're available at most five-and-dime stores.

To set: Mist your hair with setting lotion. Begin anywhere and roll up one section of hair at a time from ends to scalp. After your hair dries, take out the rollers, then brush lightly.

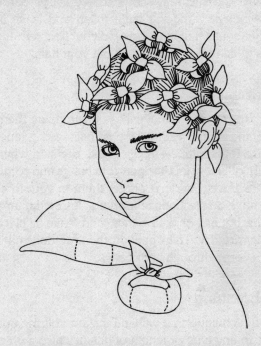

If you don't want to buy soft rollers, you can borrow a trick from Grandma's day. Make your own rollers out of soft clean cotton rags cut into strips seven or eight inches long. Place a section of dampened hair in the center of the rag, then roll up and tie closed. Continue this way until all of your hair is set.

Ponytail Pizzazz

To add body to long hair or to fluff it out when it's gone limp, try this ponytail trick. How to: Bend from the waist and brush your hair forward from nape to crown. Then gather all of your hair into a ponytail at the crown and secure it with a coated elastic band. Roll the ponytail under a large roller, and leave in place for about a half hour. Unwind your hair, remove the elastic, lightly comb or brush out your hair.

Tape Down

If your bangs bob up unevenly, you can make them behave and lie flat with a strip of hair-setting tape. Don't use regular tape—it can irritate the skin when you pull it off. How to: Dampen your bangs and comb them into place, but don't plaster them to your forehead. Leave a little bounce in them. Apply the tape along the bottom of your bangs, and leave in place until they are dry. Then peel off the tape and run a brush or comb through your bangs.

Back Brushing

Here's a technique that will add instant volume and bounce to any type or length of hair. It's also a great way to finish off your hair after you've set it. How to: Bend from the waist and brush your hair from nape to crown. Then flip it back in place and just shake into shape, or go over it gently with a brush. Do not try this trick on wet hair. Wet hair is fragile, and brushing can break it.

Finger Teasing

Finger teasing adds body and fullness to all types and lengths of hair, but works especially well on wavy or curly locks. It's gentle on the hair and won't cause snarls. How to: Slip a strand of hair between your index and middle fingers and gently slide your fingers up and down. That's all there is to it. You can finger tease here and there to fluff out portions of your hair that have fallen flat, or all over to make curly hair look twice as thick.

5

GIVE YOUR HAIR A NEW TWIST

Are you tired of wearing your hair the same old way? There are many ways you can make it look new and different for day or night. There are braids, twists, turns, roll-ups, chignons, and other styles that are fast and simple to do. All of them work best on hair that's clean and well conditioned. No special equipment is necessary. You'll need a comb, brush, coated elastic bands, bobby pins or hair pins, and a misting bottle. You might also want to set your hair first to give it more body or curl. Once you try a few of these tricks, you'll probably have some super styling ideas of your own.

PONYTAIL UPDATE

A ponytail can be pretty no matter what length of hair you have—long, medium and, yes, even short. And there's no better style when you want to keep your cool during hot weather. But first, a word of caution: Try not to wear your hair in a ponytail every day—it can cause a receding hairline or breakage. You should alternate styles to give your hair a rest. Here are some variations on the old favorite:

● For a soft romantic look, gather all of your hair to one side and pull it into a loose ponytail using a coated elastic band. Leave some tendrils free around your face. To conceal the band, pull out a section of hair from the tail you've just made and wrap it around the elastic band, tucking the ends under it. Try gathering your hair into a high side ponytail over one ear. Twist on some ribbon or cord to cover the elastic band. If your hair is very long and thick, a small ponytail placed high on the side of the head, with the rest of your hair left free, is a great variation.

• To update a classic ponytail and make it look twice as thick, pull all of your hair back into a crescent-shaped clip. Hair clips come in a variety of colors and designs, and you can pick them up in most five-and-dime stores.

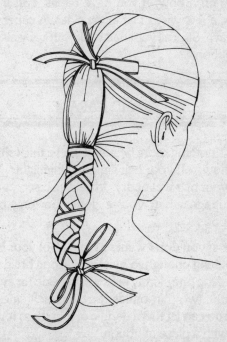

• Two ponytails are more fun than one. The trick: Gather the hair at the sides and top of your head into one ponytail and secure it with a coated elastic band. Wrap on some cord or ribbon to cover the band. Next gather the hair at the nape into a second ponytail. With a long thin piece of ribbon, tie the end of the top pony-tail to the bottom one, crisscrossing the ribbon around your hair until you reach the bottom. Then tie it. Or, instead of winding the ribbon around your hair, tie the two tails together with a series of small bows.

● A ponytail can jazz up short hair too. How to: Pull your hair back into a tiny tail at the nape of the neck and tie on a bow. If you have bangs, fluff them up, leaving a few wisps free at the sides. A super trick for the beach: Slick all your hair back with baby oil, then tie on a ribbon.

 # BRAID PARADE

There's nothing more beautiful than a thick shiny plait that shows off your hair's natural highlights. You can braid your hair wet or dry. A braid also serves as great camouflage when you've gone too long between shampoos.

● If you don't want to braid all of your hair, or if it's not long enough to twist into a long braid in back, try making one skinny braid on the side for every day. Or make two thin braids, one on each side of your face. You can let them dangle or join them together in back with a piece of ribbon.

● To dress up straight, medium-length hair, try making a whole series of braids on one side. Be sure to leave a little slack at the hairline so your hair falls softly around your face. If you alternate the lengths of the braids and space them out, they'll look more natural and blend in with the rest of your hair. For an interesting effect, try braiding in some colored or wooden beads.

• To make a single classic braid look up to date, braid it loosely. Try braiding your hair to one side so that the bottom part falls smoothly over one shoulder. Leaving some tendrils around your face and at the nape of the neck will give you a casual undone look.

• A new way to wear braids if your hair is very long: on the double. Here's how: To form two overlapping braids, first section off the hair from the crown and sides and make a braid. Then gather together the hair that's left over at the back of your head and make another braid underneath the first. Tie the braid ends with cord or ribbon.

• If your hair is medium to shoulder length, section off the hair at the crown and sides and form a single braid at the back of your head. Comb out the bottom section of your hair beneath the braid so that it forms a smooth shiny background for your plait.

• If you like to wear your hair in two classic braids that hang side by side, you can make them look snappier by tying them together at the top or bottom with a piece of ribbon or cord.

• When you want your hair to look extra special, Ralph Formisano, hairstylist at Bumble & Bumble Salon, New York City, suggests a French braid. It's

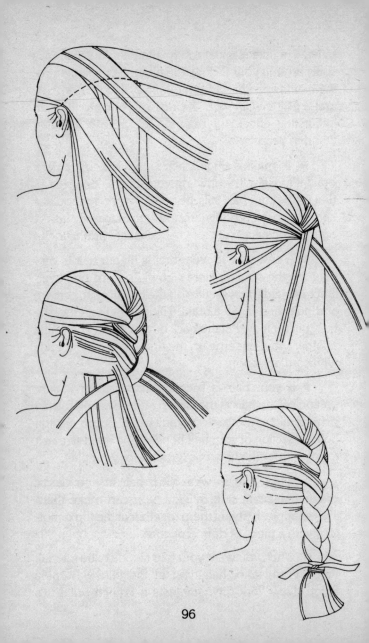

thicker and flatter than a regular braid, and lies closer to the head. It's somewhat tricky to do, but you'll catch on with a little practice. You can make just one braid or two. Here's how to make one at center back: Part your hair from the top of each ear, all the way across the back of your head. Divide the section into three parts and begin braiding. After about three turns, start weaving in small sections of hair from the left, then the right side until there's no loose hair left to take in. Finish braiding and secure the tail end with a pipe cleaner.

• To make two French braids, begin by parting your hair down the back from crown to nape. On one side, separate a section of hair about two inches thick from hairline to part. Braid it, gradually working in extra sections of hair from either side, keeping the braid close to the head. When you've finished the braid, secure the tail with a coated elastic band and repeat the process on the other side. You can let your braids dangle, or twist them into a single knot and secure with bobby pins.

• Here's Ralph's beautiful variation on the double French braid. Begin as described above, but this time add extra hair only from the section closest to the ear until there is no more left to take in. Then braid as usual using hair from center back. Secure the finished braid with a coated elastic and braid the other side the same way. Next, fold under the tail end of each braid and draw them to the back of your head and secure with bobby pins. The effect will be one continuous braid.

With just a few twists, you can add pizzazz to just about any hairstyle. Dampen your hair slightly first to make twisting easier. If you have bangs, comb them forward to keep them out of your way while you're working. When you're done, you can comb them into place and they'll be a nice contrast to the twists.

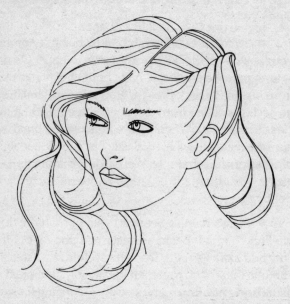

• Twist the side sections of your hair up and away from the face for several turns and secure with colorful combs. If your hair is fine, use combs with narrow-spaced teeth. For thick hair, combs with wider teeth work best. If you have trouble keeping combs in place, secure each twist with a bobby pin first, then place a comb directly in front of the bobby pin to conceal it.

● Here is a pretty look for summer or a special night out. Twist just one side of your hair and let the rest go free. Secure the twist with a few hairpins and conceal them with a piece of ribbon or cord.

● Make a thin twist on each side and join them at the back of your head. Clip with a barrette.

● This is Ralph's special style for shoulder-length to long hair. Separate a section of hair from temple to ear on each side. Twist each section all the way to the end. When you've finished twisting, the sections should resemble two pieces of rope. Next bring both sections around to the back of your head and overlap them as you would if you were braiding your hair. Secure the ends with a coated elastic band. The result will be a single ropelike twist down the back with the rest of your hair flowing free. If you like, you can coil the twist into a knot and pin in place with hair pins or bobby pins.

● Here's another look for long hair: Gather your hair together in back to form a ponytail and secure it with a coated elastic band. Twist the tail into a springy coil and wrap on another coated elastic at the bottom. Wind on some ribbon to conceal the elastics.

THE ROLL-UP

Hair rolling works best on hair that's medium to long and creates a charming, old-fashioned look. It is similar to twisting, but the rolls are looser, fuller, and rounder than twists. For the hair to be rolled easily, it must be all one length or cut in long layers. Just follow these steps.

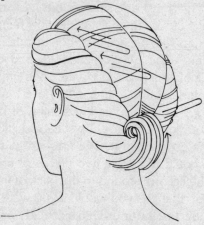

1. Part your hair down the center in back from crown to nape.

2. Starting at the temple on one side, separate a section of hair and twist it loosely up and away from the face to form a plump roll. The number of twists it takes to form a roll depends upon the length and thickness of your hair. If your hair is fine and medium length, you may only have to twist it twice to form a roll; long thick hair may have to be twisted several times to make a roll. Secure the inside of the roll to your scalp with a large bobby pin. You will have a tail of hair left over.

3. Pick up a section of hair below the one you've just rolled. Twist it and form a roll the same way as above, working in the tail from the first section. Pin

the roll with a bobby pin. Continue rolling and pinning the hair in consecutive sections until you reach the nape. Let the tail from the last section hang loose for the moment; you'll come back to it later.

4. Now roll the other side of your hair, pinning each section as you go. When you've finished, you'll have another tail left over.

5. Roll both tails over your fingers as if you were forming a pin curl and pin through the roll. If there are any gaps between the sections where the rolls join, go over them lightly with a comb, moving upward from the nape, to blend hair over them. The rolls should look smooth and seamless. If one of the rolled sections looks uneven, take it out and reroll it. You don't have to redo all of your hair to fix one uneven section.

Tip: With long hair, you can roll each side of your hair continuously, without separating it into sections.

 ## KNOTTING OPTIONS

Is your hair long or shoulder length? There are many ways to wear it up. Sweep it into a soft topknot, form it into a chignon, or knot it up at the sides. Before you start, mist your hair with water or setting lotion to smooth down stray hairs.

• It's easy to make a classic chignon. Brush out your hair and gather it into a low ponytail at the nape of the neck, using a coated elastic band. Now twist the ponytail into a rope and coil it around the base of the ponytail in a clockwise direction, securing it with bobby pins as you go. Keep coiling the ponytail to the end. You've now formed a chignon. Tuck the leftover end of the ponytail under the chignon and pin in place with bobby pins. Mist your hair lightly with hairspray to smooth down wisps.

Tip: You can vary this style by making a double chignon. Part your hair down the middle in back and form two chignons low on the nape of the neck.

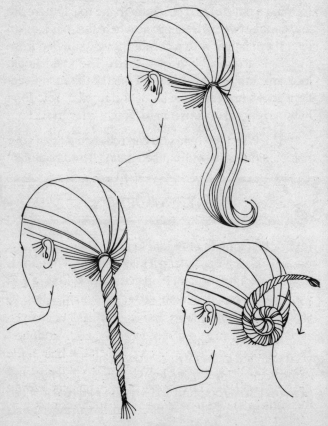

● To make a topknot, bend over and brush all of your hair forward. Hold it loosely in one hand, and catch it into a ponytail with the other. Anchor it a few inches above the scalp with a coated elastic band.

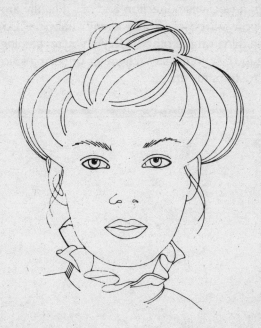

This will fluff out the hair softly. Do not twist the pony-tail—just wind it around its base to form a knot and pin securely in place with bobby pins. When you're winding your hair into a topknot, it doesn't have to be neat as a pin. You want it to look soft and "undone." For a change of pace, you can sweep the hair at the crown and sides into a topknot and leave the rest of the hair free. If you have wavy or curly hair, try leaving the ends of the knot unpinned for a tousled look.

• For double knots, divide your hair into two sections by parting it down the center from crown to nape. Brush out one half and form into a ponytail high on the side of the head, above ear level. Now twist the tail in a clockwise direction and coil it tightly around the ponytail base. Secure it with hairpins. Do the same thing on the other side. As you're winding, be sure to mist your hair with water or setting lotion to control the stray ends.

6

SNAPPY
HAIR
ACCESSORIES

Hair ornaments are more popular than ever now, so when you want to make your hair look special in a flash, add one on. Many of the accessories that you see in stores are made from materials you probably have right at home. Check out your jewelry box, dresser drawers, or attic trunks for pretty trinkets that can double as hair accessories. Your search might turn up some finds that are much more original than anything you could buy—and a lot cheaper, too. A long scarf, a strip of fancy fabric, a piece of lace, a length of satiny cord, even a necktie make attractive hair accessories. Save ribbons and bows from holiday and birthday presents; almost anything that sparkles or shines will look wonderful in your hair. The slim gold cording on some packages, for instance, makes a super headband.

Notions stores carry all kinds of small treasures that you can fashion into hair accessories. You'll find satin and grosgrain ribbons in all widths, fake flowers, feathers, glittery strips of sequin-covered fabric, bogus pearls, and beads. For nighttime wear there are shimmery metallic ribbons or thin cording in silver or gold.

HOW TO WEAR HAIR ORNAMENTS

There are dozens of ways to dress up your hair with accessories. A pair of pretty combs or barrettes anchored behind your ears can make all the difference. Or just sweep one side of your hair back with a comb. If your hair isn't long enough to hold a comb, you can use bobby pins—plain or fancy—to tuck your hair behind your ears. Headbands add interest to any hairstyle—long, short, medium, or layered. You can also twist a scarf or bandanna and tie it on as a headband or wear it Indian-style. A slim necktie is another bright headband idea. Tie it on and let the ends dangle.

If you have a lot of hair to work with, you can wear bold accessories. Try twisting a scarf and tying it into a fluffy bow. For a sporty look, you can pull your hair back into a ponytail, then twist a scarf or a piece of soft leather or fabric around it. An attention-getting trick: Twist pieces of hair at random all over your head and clip on small colorful barrettes.

To jazz up your hair for evening, there are lots of fun effects you can create with accessories. For an eye-catching headband, twist a sparkly scarf or a piece of fabric and tie it on any way you like—hide the knot in back or let it show at the side or top of your head. You can wind a strand of pearls or beads around a chignon or pierce the chignon with an ornamental chopstick. Tuck flowers or feathers into twisted lengths of hair.

For all-out dazzle, mist your hair with setting lotion and sprinkle on some glitter or shimmery metallic powder. It will wash out in your next shampoo. Or try a smattering of tiny gold or silver stick-on stars. You can even use tinfoil to make your hair look special. Here's how: Wrap thin strands of hair with small strips of foil. Concentrate the foil at the sides of your hair, or wrap strips of it all over your head. Vary the lengths of the also works as a hair wrapping. Starting at the scalp, knot a piece of cord around a thin section of hair and wind it down and around the strand to the end, then knot again. Do as many sections as you like.

Other accessories can complement the ornaments you wear in your hair. If you sweep your hair off your face with a headband or put your hair up, beautiful earrings will enhance the effect. If you're wearing a simple hair ornament, wear more daring earrings. One long, dangling earring will look more dramatic than a matching pair, especially if you're wearing your hair all to one side. If your hair is short, clip it back with small barrettes or bobby pins and finish off the look with small stud earrings—pearls, leaf designs, rhinestones, or gemstones will all look nice. Having your ears pierced is something to consider if your hair is short—there's nothing prettier than sparkly earrings peeking out from beneath wispy layers of hair.

Makeup can also work as an accessory to complement your hairstyle. For day, soft peaches and pinks for cheeks and lips are flattering on just about everyone. Just make sure to keep blusher and lipstick in the same color family. Taupe, gray, fawn, apricot, or celery green shadow will play up your eyes without being overpowering. For night, you can go for richer, more vibrant colors—gentle rose or spicy peach for cheeks; burgundy, cinnamon, or burnished coral for lips. Go all out with eye shadow after dark, too. Smoky blue, heathery violet, deep teal, bronze, and copper are shades you might want to try. To make your eyes really sparkle, highlight your browbones strips for an interesting effect. Thin gold or silver cord (the area directly beneath your eyebrows) with a light dusting of gold eyeshadow.

Keep in mind that cool shades of makeup such as pink, rose, blue, and gray will look prettiest with silver accessories. Warm colors like peach, brown, coral, sienna, and nutmeg complement gold or bronze accessories. All of your accessories, in fact— hair ornaments, makeup, and earrings—should work together, harmonize. One accessory should not cancel out another one, or overpower the clothes you're wearing. For example, if you have on a dramatic headband, you might want to wear small earrings or skip them altogether. But if you have just a sliver of something in your hair, your earrings can be bolder.

A foolproof way to check the effect you've created is to take a long look in a full-length mirror when you're completely dressed. If you're in doubt about any item, take it off. That goes for makeup too. If you suspect you might have overdone it, tone it down. You can remove excess eye makeup with a dampened cotton swab. If your blusher looks too bright, take some of it off with a cotton ball.

Keep your accessories in the same mood as your clothes, too. Satin ribbons and bows are romantic and look nicest with soft feminine clothes. Chamois and leather hair ornaments will look great with your jeans. Black and red accessories are always right for night. Silver, gold, and bronze are effective anytime. One of the newest looks is to wear metallic accessories during the day. A bronze headband, clip, or set of combs will look sensational worn with casual skirts, pants, and sweaters.

DESIGN YOUR OWN

It doesn't take much money to make your own hair accessories—just a little time and imagination. Here are complete instructions on how to make you own creations. Pick up a container of fabric glue such as Sobo; you'll need it to paste ornaments onto headbands, combs, and barrettes.

Combs

Hair combs are the simplest accessories to decorate. The most common ones are plastic tortoiseshell. Most five-and-dime stores carry them. The brim of the comb, the part above the teeth, is the place to put the trimmings. You can glue on a frothy piece of lace, a spray of tiny fake flowers, rows of rickrack, or strips of ribbon in contrasting colors. Trinkets such as little hearts or moons or tiny seashells that you've collected on the beach all make beautiful decorations. A trim of feathers is flirty and fun. Make creative combinations—ribbons plus shells or lace mixed with flowers. If you want something flashier, glue feathers over a strip of glittery fabric.

For the best results, plan your design before you begin. Then when you're ready to go to work, cut the piece of fabric or ribbon a bit longer than the comb. Coat the wrong side of the fabric with glue and press it

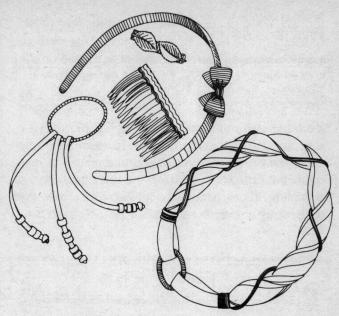

down, smoothing it out to remove any bulges. Put a drop of glue on the ends of the fabric and fold them around to the back of the comb. You won't be able to see them when the combs are in your hair.

To paste on a trinket, smear a small amount of glue on the back of it, then press it down on the comb. If some of the glue oozes out, wipe it away with a clean damp cloth. Let the glue dry for at least twenty minutes.

Ponytail Holders

Another ornament that's a cinch to make is a ponytail holder. The materials you'll need: a package of coated elastic bands from the five-and-dime store, about a foot and a half of colored cord, and some fake pearls or beads from a notions shop. Cut the cord into three six-inch strips and knot the end of each one on the coated elastic band. Slip pearls or beads onto each cord. You can use one pearl or bead per cord, or as many as you like. If you have an assortment of beads, decorate each strand differently. Knot each cord at the end and snip off the tails so there are no ends sticking out. Now you'll have three pretty streamers. This kind of holder also looks nice at the end of a braid, either a regular braid or small side braid. Another simple way to dress up a coated elastic band: Tie a big satin bow on it.

 # EASY DOES IT

In addition to combs and ponytail holders, you can make beautiful bandannas, headbands, and barrettes. The following ideas are from M.B. McCallister, a New York City designer of hair acessories. The results are as special as anything you'll find in a store, and unbelievably easy to achieve. Once you master the basic designs, you can go on to make your own original hair ornaments.

Bandannas

Bandannas are the hottest new hair accessories. This one can be worn as a regular headband or as a browband. Materials: a piece of fabric cut into a twelve-inch square, a yard of ribbon, and a two-inch strip of elastic. Instead of fabric, you can use a bandanna from the dime store if you like. The Western-style ones look snappiest and come in bright colors like red, turquoise, and purple.

Directions: Twist the fabric tightly until it looks like a rope. Clamp one end with a clothespin to keep it from unraveling and have a friend hold the other end or hold it between your knees. Next, clamp one end of the ribbon under the clothespin with the fabric. Holding the fabric taut, wind the ribbon around it.

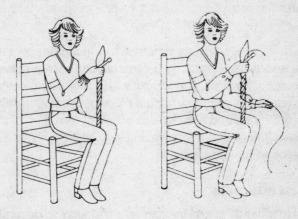

When you reach the end, cut the ribbon and turn it with the end of the fabric under, forming a loop. Glue or stitch in place. Now remove the clothespin and form a loop at the other end the same way. Use any leftover ribbon to conceal the glued or stitched portions of the bandanna. Just spread some glue on the wrong side of a small piece of ribbon and wind it around one end of the bandanna, just above the loop. Do the same thing on the other end. The last step:

Slip the piece of elastic through the loops and stitch closed. This will let the band stretch when you put it on.

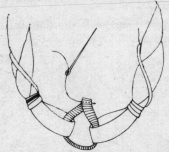

There are countless variations on this design. For a sporty headband, you can substitute thick cotton cording for fabric and wrap it with a bright strip of terrycloth. For evening, wind a piece of sparkly metallic cording around a thick piece of satiny cord. For a fancier bandanna, try wrapping two ribbons or cords around the base layer.

Headbands

Headbands are so inexpensive and easy to decorate that you can have a different one for every day of the week. Materials: a plastic headband from the five-and-dime store and a piece of satin, velvet, or grosgrain ribbon slightly wider than your headband.

Directions: Cut two strips of ribbon that are two inches longer than the headband. Put the wrong sides of the ribbon together, and machine stitch the edges lengthwise to make a casing. Now slip the casing over the band and center it so that it's about an inch longer

114

than the band on each side. Turn under the raw edges of the casing on each side and glue them to the inside of the band. Clamp clothespins over the raw edges to help set the glue. Let dry for twenty minutes.

The way you decorate your headband is up to you. Some suggestions: You can make a bow out of ribbon and glue it on one side of the band or make a whole slew of tiny ribbons and glue them across the top. Metallic ribbons are pretty for evening. Another option: rhinestones. Place one rhinestone slightly off-center at the top of the band for a sleek, elegant look. Or you can sprinkle rhinestones along the entire length of the band. To secure a rhinestone, place a drop of glue on the back of it, then press it onto the band. Avoid using metallic or satin ribbon as a head-band covering if you want to use rhinestones as decorations; they won't adhere very well. Use cotton or velvet instead.

Barrettes

Here's a design for a barrette that's so beautiful that all you need is one. For materials you'll need a thin, flat, metal barrette available at the five-and-dime store, two small leaves made of wire and covered with net or fabric, and a strip of satin ribbon eight inches long and a quarter of an inch wide. You may have net or fabric leaves at home, left over from holiday or birthday gifts. If not, you can pick them up for pennies at a novelty shop.

How to: Twist the stems of the two leaves around the top portion of the barrette so that the tips of the leaves meet in the center. To cover the stems, wrap the barrette with satin ribbon. When you get to a leaf, lift it up and wind the ribbon underneath it. Glue each end of the ribbon to the back of the barrette.

7

SPORTS
STYLE

Anything that's good for your health is good for your hair. Regular exercise benefits your whole body by revving up your circulatory system. Once the blood gets moving, it circulates right up to the scalp where it nourishes the hair root that makes your hair grow.

 ## HAIR HASSLES

There's no doubt about it. Sports are super for your hair. But playing them everyday presents special hair-care problems.

If you lead a sporting life, your hair needs special care. Constant exposure to sun, wind, and salt water can be harsh on your hair. Pool chemicals such as chlorine can damage it; humid weather can frazzle it. Here are the most common hair problems you're likely to encounter if you're active in sports, and tips on how to correct them—from hair expert Bets Bisceglia for Glemby at Bloomingdale's in New York City.

• SNARLS Nothing feels nicer than the wind whipping through your hair when you're whizzing along on your bike or playing games outside. The problem is, your hair may be a mass of snarls afterward. If you tug and pull at your hair to get the snarls out, you may be left with an even bigger problem: split ends. Or, if you rip at the hair with a comb or brush, you risk tearing it out by the roots. Here's the right way to remove snarls. With a wide-tooth comb, gently comb the underlayers of your hair first. Starting at the nape of the neck, separate a small section and comb through it, lifting the rest of the hair up and out of the way. If you encounter a knot, work it out gently with your fingers. Continue combing your hair in small section from the bottom up until you reach the crown. Then move on to the sides and do the same thing. Now comb your hair from crown to nape—it should be free of tangles.

- DRYNESSS The sun can sap your hair of oil, leaving it dry and, in extreme cases, brittle. The sun's ultraviolet rays are what are causing the damage, and they're much more intense when reflected off a surface like a sandy beach. In summer the damaging effects of the sun are compounded by salt water, which also dries out the hair. To protect your hair, comb some instant conditioner through it, then slick it back. It will look pretty this way if you tie it back with a ribbon. It's also a good idea to keep your hair covered with a hat or scarf during prolonged exposure to the sun. This is especially true if you have a perm—it can easily turn into frizz during the summer. If your hair feels sticky after swimming in salt water, carry along a small misting bottle filled with fresh water and spray your hair to remove some of the salt.

- CHLORINE Chlorine is another culprit—it leaves hair dry and lackluster. In addition, too much copper in the water can impart a greenish cast to the hair—usually only noticeable on blonds. If you swim every day, it's essential to step up your hair-care routine. Before you go into the pool, work some instant conditioner or creme rinse into your hair to protect it. And always wear a bathing cap. Bathing caps don't have to be unattractive. You can find lightweight racing caps in shocking colors like pink and yellow.

When you come out of the pool, shampoo and condition your hair, then try this trick: Rinse your hair with apple cider vinegar. There's probably a bottle of it in your kitchen cabinet. It will remove any chemical residue from your hair and leave it sparkling clean and shiny. If your hair is oily, you can use the vinegar straight. For normal to dry hair, dilute one ounce of it in about three ounces of water. Pour the mixture through the hair, then rinse out. You can use the vinegar rinse about twice a week—any more than that can dry out your hair. If your hair is dry to the point of brittleness, a hot oil treatment will help restore moisture and sheen.

- STATIC ELECTRICITY This is usually only a problem during the winter, when cold dry air can strip your hair of moisture. And overheated air indoors only makes the problem worse. Rx: Use an instant conditioner after every shampoo, without fail. To prevent your hair from becoming dry and therefore more susceptible to static, keep it covered. This is especially important on the ski slopes where the sun's rays are even stronger than they are on the beach. And brush your hair every night before you go to bed to distribute the oils.

- FRIZZIES Humid or damp weather, or perspiration caused by vigorous activity, may set off a case of the frizzies. But you can beat them just by using a setting lotion before you exercise. Use a liquid rather than a gel, and choose one made for your type of hair. Or use lemon juice, which works especially well on oily hair. Just squeeze a lemon, strain the juice, and comb it through your hair. If your hair is naturally curly or permed, let it dry naturally. Blowdry straight hair. In addition to taming your frizzies, setting lotions have other bonuses that make them ideal for sports. They coat the hair somewhat to protect it from the sun and give it body and direction so it won't hang down in your face during a game. Setting lotions will make your hair wonderfully shiny, too. You might want to try putting some on even if you don't have the frizzies.

● OILINESS Depending on the sport you play and the time of year, your scalp may become oilier than normal. Keeping your hair covered with a hat during winter sports can make the scalp sweat and also stimulate oil production. So can warm weather. To combat oiliness, wash your hair as often as you like, even a couple of times a day if you feel you need to. Use just a small amount of shampoo or dilute it with water to prevent your hair from drying out. Then follow up with an instant conditioner to restore moisture. If your hair is oily at the roots and dry at the ends, try this remedy: Massage your scalp first. Then saturate a cotton ball with witch hazel, which is a mild astringent. Dab your entire scalp with it to whisk away oils and to dislodge any flakes. Then shampoo your hair and condition it as usual.

There's nothing easier to maintain than short hair if sports are a part of your everyday routine. A cropped cut that you can just fluff dry is real bliss. But short hair isn't the only answer if you're sports-minded. Any basic hairstyle that you can wash and wear will work beautifully. It can be long, medium, or short, just as long as it doesn't require setting or spending lots of time coaxing into shape with a blowdrier.

If your hair refuses to behave after a few hours of activity, you may need a new cut. Tell your stylist that you need a carefree cut that requires minimal upkeep. And don't fight your natural hair texture—by blowdrying curly hair into a straight style, for instance. It just won't hold its shape after a hard game of tennis or a dip in the pool. If your hair starts to wilt, and hangs in your face as soon as the action gets hot on the court or playing field, try one of these super sports styles created by Bets Bisceglia for Glemby at Bloomingdale's. Whether your hair is short or long, there's a style to suit you.

Short to Chin-Length Hair

If your hair is short to chin length, the best way to keep it off your face is with a sweatband or bandanna in an absorptive material such as terrycloth or cotton. Sweatbands are available at sporting goods stores, or you can make your own out of a strip of stretchy terry-cloth. Or use a cotton bandanna from the dime store. Twist the bandanna into a taut rope, slip it on over your head as you would a headband, and knot it at the nape of your neck. Or tie it on Indian-style across your forehead, making sure not to tie it on too tightly or your hair will bulge out over it.

Medium to Long Hair

The following style will keep your hair in place beautifully. You're going to form two tight coils of hair along the hairline on each side of the head and then join them together at the nape of the neck. How to:

1. First divide your hair into two sections by parting it from crown to nape at the center back of your head. Grasp one section of hair in your hand and hold it up behind your ear.

2. Begin twisting the hair up and back away from the face to form a tight coil. Twist the hair in one continuous motion all the way down to the nape, keeping the coil close to the hairline. There will be a small tail of hair left over at the end.

3. Have a friend hold the coil you've just made while you twist the other side of your hair the same way. You'll have another tail left over at the end of the coil.

4. Join the two coils together at the nape, using a coated elastic band. Wrap on some cord or ribbon to cover the elastic band. A ponytail will hang below the coiled hair. You don't have to have a long ponytail left over to wear this style. A small tail will look just fine.

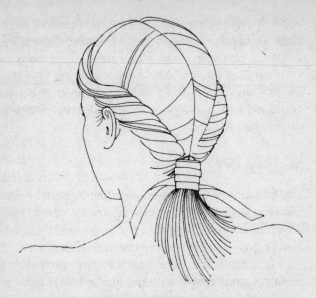

Variations: If you have a fairly long ponytail left over after you've secured the coils with the coated elastic, pick up the tail, roll the ends under toward the scalp, and clamp with a barrette. Or try twisting the ponytail into a coil, too, and secure it at the bottom with a coated elastic band. Wrap on some ribbon or cord to cover the band.

Long to Very Long Hair

The following sensational styles will keep your hair under control during all but the most rigorous sports. They're based on a simple system of ponytails, but there are lots of variations. Once you know where to put the ponytails, you can braid, tuck, and twist your hair anyway you like. Just be sure to use coated elastic bands to secure the hair, and to leave a little slack when you pull it back. Here's a step-by-step styling guide.

1. Part your hair above each ear, straight around to the back of your head. Gather the hair together, comb it out and secure it in a ponytail just below the crown.

2. Part the rest of your hair down the middle. Gather up the hair on one side and form another ponytail, making sure it rests close to the part at the back of your head. Do the same thing on the other side. These two ponytails should line up evenly and be fairly close together.

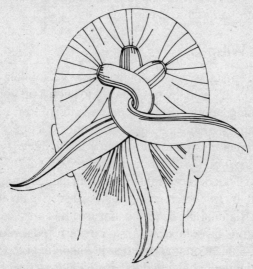

3. Now overlap the side ponytails as if you were starting to braid. Include the top ponytail in with them, and braid until you come to the end. Tie with a coated elastic band, or tuck the ends of the hair under at the nape and secure with a barrette.

Variations: This is a pretty look for a dance class. Gather the side ponytails together and twist twice. Twist the crown ponytail in with them, then coil the hair into a knot and secure with bobby pins. If your hair is very thick, make four ponytails. Form the first ponytail the same as above, then part your hair down the center in back. To make a side ponytail, gather up the hair behind one ear and make a ponytail close to the part, leaving some hair free at the nape. Do the same thing on the other side. Form the fourth ponytail with the hair at the nape. You can now braid or twist your hair as you like.

Sports Wrap-Up

Head wrapping is one of the newest looks for hair of any length. It's also the perfect way to keep it off your face during sports, and to protect it from sun and wind damage. Here's a basic wrap-up that's open to many variations. It's so pretty that you'll want to try it even when you're off the court or playing field.

You'll need a scarf that's thirty-four inches square or a forty by sixty-inch rectangle. Use a scarf in an absorbent material like cotton so that your hair and scalp can breathe. If you're using a square scarf, fold it into a triangle. Place it on your head as if you were going to tie it under your chin, but don't. Instead, draw the corners of the scarf behind your head and cross them at the nape. Now twist each corner into a taut rope. Raise the corners of the scarf up to the top of your

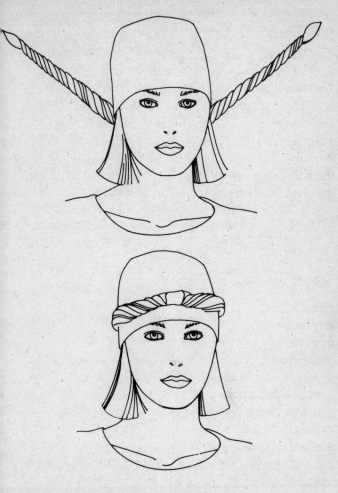

head and tie them together in a knot. Tuck the leftover flap in at the nape. If you use a rectangular scarf, it's not necessary to fold it; just put it on as above, twist the ends, and tie at the crown.

8

COLOR
BOOSTERS

Just as no one is really satisfied with the type of hair she has, most of us wish we were born with a more exciting hair color. Girls with black hair long to be blond, brunets think their hair color is boring, blonds want to go lighter, brighter. The truth is, there's no such thing as a dull hair color. If you wash and condition your hair regularly, eat wholesome foods, and get the proper amount of rest and exercise, your hair will look healthy and shiny. And if you'd like to heighten your natural highlights, or experiment with color, you can do it without damaging your hair by using the color boosters coming up in this chapter.

In general, it's not advisable to change the color of your hair in a big way until you're out of your teens. Colors produced by dyes and tints can look unnatural on you. This is the time to make the most of your natural beauty.

If you do want a dramatic color change, be aware that many hair-coloring products contain strong chemicals that can damage your hair over time. You may also become a slave to your hair. You'll have to retouch the roots and pay special attention to conditioning because dyes can dry out your hair, make it dull and brittle. And even though many advertisers claim that their products are foolproof and easy to apply, if you're inexperienced at using them you may wind up with a color you didn't bargain for. After you've colored your hair, you're stuck with that shade until it grows out. There's no way to switch back to your natural hair color without putting more chemicals on your hair.

The hair-coloring products to avoid are semipermanent and permanent dyes and tints, many of which come in shampoo-in formulas. Semipermanent dyes coat the hair and intensify or deepen the color, but won't lighten it. This type of color lasts up to four or six weeks and fades with each shampoo. But after repeated applications, the dye can build up on the hair ends and look unnatural.

Permanent dyes and tints can lighten or darken the hair, producing a marked color change. The dye penetrates to the innermost layer of the hairshaft to change the pigment. Repeated use can dull and dry out the hair, making it more prone to breakage. This kind of color is for keeps—you have to live with it until it grows out completely. If you lighten your hair, you will have to retouch the roots every three to four weeks.

 ## NATURAL HAIR SHINERS

If you want to add highlights to your hair, you don't have to use chemical dyes. There are many natural rinses you can use that will make your hair glisten and gleam. Wash your hair and rinse it as usual, then use one of the following gentle hair shiners. (Unless otherwise noted, leave the solution on your hair for a few minutes, then lightly rinse it out. If you don't have some of the herbal ingredients on hand, you can pick them up at a health food store.)

• LEMON JUICE   Lemon juice is a natural hair lightener. It brightens up all shades of hair but works best on light brown or blond hair. Mix one part lemon juice with eight parts water and pour it through your hair. Make sure to use fresh lemon juice. The bottled kind may contain preservatives which can give a greenish cast to blond hair. Another thing you can do is squeeze the juice of one lemon on your hair full strength and sit in the sun. The lemon juice hastens the natural lightening action of the sun and creates beautiful highlights. After a few hours, rinse and then shampoo your hair.

• APPLE CIDER VINEGAR   Both lemon juice and apple cider vinegar restore the hair's natural acid mantle and smooth down the cuticle so your hair looks its glossiest. In addition, apple cider vinegar deep-cleans your hair by removing every last trace of shampoo. (Soapy residue can leave a dull film on the hair.) The recipe: one part vinegar to eight parts water.

• PARSLEY   Parsley was once thought to prevent loss of hair, but what it really does is give a glorious sheen to the hair. To make a parsley rinse, put two tablespoons of fresh parsley leaves in a pint of boiling water, let the infusion steep, then strain. After the mixture cools, pour it through your hair.

• CHAMOMILE   The sweet-smelling flowers from the chamomile gently lighten blond hair. A chamomile rinse can also be used to even out the tones in blond hair that's been bleached by the sun and is coming in darker at the roots. Add two tablespoons of the dried chamomile flowers to a pint of boiling water, or make a strong brew of chamomile tea, using two to three tea bags, and let steep. Strain if necessary, and pour over your hair when cool.

• ORANGE PEKOE TEA   Orange pekoe tea, an ordinary household tea, will add a burnished glow to light or dark brown hair. Brew up a strong pot using two to three tea bags, let cool, and pour through the hair.

• ROSEMARY   Over the ages, rosemary has been used as a cure-all. It makes dark hair come alive, helps prevent dandruff, and smells heavenly. Add two tablespoons of rosemary to a pint of boiling water, let steep, and strain. When cool, pour on and work through to the ends of the hair.

• NETTLE   This prickly plant brightens any shade of hair. It adds body, too. Simmer two tablespoons of nettles in a pint of boiling water. Strain, let cool, then rinse through the hair.

• RED ZINGER TEA   It's one of the best ways to rev up red hair. Add two tablespoons of tea to a pint of boiling water and let steep. Squeeze in the juice of a lemon and rinse through the hair. Sit in the sun and let dry. Then rinse and shampoo the hair.

• SAFFRON   Saffron adds a radiant reddish glow to light or dark brown hair. Add a pinch to a cup of boiling water, stir, and let cool. Then pour through the hair.

Tip: Herbs aren't for rinses only. To help control an oily or flaky scalp, put a tablespoon or two of thyme into a cup of boiling water and let steep. After the mixture cools, add it to your shampoo or conditioner.

Here are some fast ways to change the color of your hair temporarily. They're all simple and safe, so experiment and have fun. Try more than one!

• TEMPORARY RINSES   Temporary rinses come in all shades from blond to black and can enrich your hair color, but won't lighten it. Some come premixed; others must be diluted in boiling water. A temporary rinse lets you play with color, without locking you into a shade. You can wash it out right away if you don't like it. If you're pleased with the way your hair comes out, you can find temporary rinses that last through three shampoos.

• SPRAY-ON HIGHLIGHTS   Spray-on highlights are colors that come in an aerosol container. Spray on some gold streaks, add red highlights, or go all out and try a crazy shade like fuchsia—hot stuff on black hair. Spray on designs such as stripes or stars. The color comes out the next time you wash your hair.

• INSTANT COLOR   All you need is some powder blush or eyeshadow in a sparkly shade to wake up your hair color. Mist your hair with setting lotion first. Then dust on some highlights using a small paintbrush. Some suggestions: Try coppery blush on brown hair for a burnished effect, or coral blush on blond hair for strawberry-blond lights. To make black hair shimmer, use silvery shadow as a hair highlighter. Liven up red with a dusting of golden blush or shadow.

HENNA

Henna is a vegetable dye that has been used for centuries as a hair coloring throughout the Middle East. Cleopatra is said to have used it to coat her hair to protect it from the sun.

Henna comes in powder form and is mixed with hot water before it is applied. It is available in a variety of shades such as red, light to dark brown, black, and neutral—which is colorless. The colored shades of henna add warm reddish highlights to brown and black hair. Neutral henna can be used on any shade of hair to add body and shine.

Colored henna must be used with caution. If you're not careful, your hair could turn out too red. And because henna is a dye, you'll have to live with the color until it grows out from the roots. For the best results, look for a pure natural henna containing no metallic dyes or salts, which could dry out the hair and produce an unexpected color change. Here are some tips from hairstylist Ralph Formisano of Bumble & Bumble Salon in New York City on how to choose and use the correct shade of henna.

• BROWN HAIR For natural-looking results on brown hair, use the shade of henna closest to your own hair color—light, medium, or dark brown. Then, depending upon the effect you want—highlights or a definite color change—mix a little or a lot of red henna with brown henna. For glints of red, add a tablespoon of red henna to a packet of brown henna. Equal parts of brown and red will produce a distinct color change. You can alter these proportions somewhat, but here's a good rule of thumb: The lighter your hair, the less red henna you should use. That's because red henna shows up more on light hair than on dark hair. To heighten the effects of brown and red henna, you can substitute hot coffee or orange pekoe tea for the hot water called for in the package instructions.

- BLACK HAIR If you have black hair, avoid using pure black henna. No one's hair is that dark. To give black hair a boost, use half black and half brown henna for a more natural look.
- BLOND HAIR To perk up blond hair, neutral henna is best. Try this recipe: Follow the package instructions for mixing, but instead of adding hot water to the henna powder, use chamomile tea. The henna will make the natural colorant in chamomile adhere to the hair better.

Before you apply henna, Ralph recommends giving your hair a deep conditioning treatment. For full penetration of the conditioner, cover your hair with a plastic bag or shower cap after applying it. After the specified amount of time, rinse your hair thoroughly and towel it dry before putting on henna. The henna will help seal in the conditioner.

Words to the Wise

When using colored henna, you can't always rely on package instructions to tell you how your hair will turn out, so a strand test is a must. It takes only a few minutes, and by previewing the color you can prevent disaster later on. How to: Mix a small amount of henna with water to form a paste and apply it to a few strands of hair in an unnoticeable spot—beneath the top layer of hair on the side, for instance. Leave the henna on for the same amount of time you were planning to during full application (see instructions for applying henna, coming up). Then wipe it off with a damp paper towel and check the color.

Never use henna if you've already colored your hair. It will be impossible to predict how it will react. You can have your hair permed after using it, provided your hair is in good condition, but it will take longer for the waving solution to penetrate because it has to break through the henna coating.

Applying Henna:

Here's the basic procedure to follow once you've done a strand test and you're ready to apply the henna for real. Be sure to wear rubber gloves if you're using colored henna; the dye stains the skin. Also, to ensure even application, use a wide-tooth comb or small hair-coloring brush, available at any beauty supply store.

1. Following package instructions, mix henna with hot water and stir to form a thick paste. Very important: Always mix henna in a glass or ceramic container—never a metal one.

2. After the mixture cools, comb or brush it through your hair in small sections from the roots to the ends. If the ends of your hair are dry, they'll soak

up color fastest. So, to avoid overly bright ends, wait until processing time is almost up, then comb henna through the ends of your hair.

3. When you've distributed the henna evenly through your hair, slick it back with a comb. Wrap a plastic bag over your hair or cover it with tin foil for deep penetration.

4. Leave the mixture on your hair for about fifteen to thirty minutes for highlights, or sixty minutes for a definite color change. Then rinse it out and shampoo.

Tip: Proper timing is the key to using henna successfully. The longer you leave it on your hair the more pronounced the color will be, so keep an eye on the clock after you've applied it.

 # HAIR LIGHTENERS

There are many hair lighteners available for home use, such as hair-painting kits and gentle lighteners that promise to make your hair look as if you've spent a summer in the sun. Bleach is the lightening agent in these products. Unlike temporary rinses or dyes, bleach doesn't deposit color. In fact, it does just the reverse. It strips the hair of color from inside the hairshaft.

The most common type of bleach is hydrogen peroxide. When used properly, bleach can produce very natural-looking effects, but it's hard on the hair. Repeated applications can dry out and dull the hair and overlighten it, resulting in dark roots when your hair starts to grow in.

Gentle Lighteners

According to hairstylist Ralph Formisano, gentle hair lighteners—those designed to give your hair an overall sunny glow or to be used in the sun—are for blond and light brown hair only. Why? For one thing, medium brown to dark hair has red, not gold highlights. When you bleach black hair, for example, it must go through three stages before it becomes blond— brown, red, and gold. Lighteners formulated for blond or light brown hair aren't strong enough to take darker hair beyond the middle stages. Medium brown hair will turn a brassy gold, and very dark hair will become an unnatural shade of red. But when gentle lighteners are used on light brown or blond hair, the effect is a brighter, sunnier version of the same shade.

Ralph recommends using these lighteners for the minimum amount of time specified on the package label if you want just a slight color lift. Keep in mind that your hair will become lighter and lighter every time you process it, and the sun will heighten the effect even more. If you're not careful, you could wind up a towhead when all you wanted was a few highlights.

Hair Painting

One of the simplest ways to add sunny highlights to your hair is with a hair-painting kit. You just take a brush and paint on highlights where you want them. For the most natural-looking highlights, Ralph Formisano suggests painting very thin strands around your face and at the top of the head, where the sun usually hits. He feels it's safest to do only a few strands of hair at a time because you can always paint on more, but you can't remove highlights once you have them. Aim for the shade your hair turns when you've spent time in the sun, and always do a strand test first to determine the shade.

As you paint your hair, touch the top layer only and check from time to time to see how the color is developing. To do this, wipe the bleach off a strand of hair with a damp paper towel and examine the hair in daylight if possible to make sure it isn't coming out too light. For subtle highlights, you'll want to rinse the bleach mixture out after a fairly short time. In any case, never leave the bleach on longer than the maximum time recommended on the package—usually fifteen to twenty minutes—or you could wind up with a zebra-striped effect.

Hair painting requires minimal upkeep—you'll need to do it two or three times a year at most. And, if you've highlighted your hair correctly, there won't be a telltale root line when your highlights begin to grow out. When you retouch your hair, avoid painting new highlights over old ones. This can damage your hair and look artificial. Instead, coat the old highlights with a thick conditioner to protect them from the bleach and paint in new highlights, avoiding the coated strands.

A Final Word

When using any type of hair lightener, always read the instructions carefully before starting. Wrap a towel around your shoulders to keep the bleach mixture from spattering onto your clothes. Wear rubber gloves to protect your hands, and make sure to keep the bleach out of your eyes. Never use a lightener or any other hair-coloring product if your scalp is irritated or if you've recently colored your hair. Don't bleach your hair and have a permanent the same day. Perm your hair a few weeks beforehand. After bleaching, use a shampoo formulated specially for color-treated hair, and step up your conditioning routine.

9

TROUBLE-SHOOTING GUIDE

Even the healthiest head of hair can show signs of wear and tear. Combing, brushing, and blowdrying can damage your hair to some extent. Perming, coloring, and overexposure to the elements compound hair problems. Thankfully, hair is sturdy stuff and can withstand an amazing amount of abuse. But it can take only so much before it needs first aid. Here are some of the biggest enemies of your hair and how to combat them. Some of this information has been covered in other chapters and some of it is new, but this list will sum it all up for you.

THE TEN TOP HAIR VILLAINS

• OVERWASHING Frequent shampooing is essential to maintaining shiny hair and a healthy scalp. But too much washing with a harsh shampoo can strip your hair of moisture and oil. You can shampoo your hair every day and not damage it, provided you use a mild shampoo. To test the strength of your shampoo, dab a drop on your face and leave it on for a few moments. If it stings or leaves a red mark, it's too strong and you should switch to a gentler one. Too vigorous washing is also bad for your hair—hard tugging can pull it out by the toots. Wash your hair thoroughly but gently.

• IMPROPER BRUSHING If you read the section on brushing, you know that you don't have to brush your hair a hundred strokes a day to keep it shiny. About twenty-five strokes daily is all it takes to stimulate the scalp, dislodge surface dirt, and get the oils in your hair flowing. Overbrushing can make your hair too oily, especially if you have a problem with the greasies to begin with. Make sure to use a brush with pliant bristles. Sharp bristles can scratch your scalp and break off your hair, causing split ends. Brush in long smooth strokes, not short choppy ones. Yanking a brush through your hair can rip it right out of your scalp.

- HEAT   Whether from a blowdrier or the sun, too much heat can harm your hair. Always use your blowdrier on the medium, not the hot, setting. Hold it at least six inches away from your hair, and never aim it on one spot for more than a few seconds. For more protection against blowdrying abuse, there are conditioning lotions you can put on before blowdrying to protect your hair from heat. If you spend a prolonged period of time in the sun, cover your hair with a hat or a scarf or slick on a conditioner while you're outdoors.

- POLLUTION   Soot and dust in the air make your hair dirtier faster. In addition, polluted air contains particles that can eat into the hairshaft and damage the cells. The best way to fight pollution is to keep your hair sparkling clean. If you live in a city, you'll have to wash your hair more often than if you live in a rural area.

- TOO MUCH CONDITIONING   Conditioning should be a regular part of your hair-care routine, but don't overdo it. Too much conditioning can leave a heavy coating on the hair that makes it look dull, limp, and greasy. Choose a conditioner that suits your hair type.

If your hair is fine, for instance, use a light liquid conditioner after every shampoo, not a heavy cream one. Oily hair might not need a conditioner at all. No matter what type of conditioner you use, make sure to rinse it out thoroughly.

- OVERPROCESSING Dry brittle hair that doesn't shine can be caused by a perm or straightening solution that was left on too long, or by coloring. What your hair needs is tender loving care and conditioning. Comb and brush it gently and give it frequent hot oil treatments—once a week if the damage is severe. Never perm and color your hair the same day. If you have a perm, try to wait until all of it has grown out before you have another one. If you've straightened your hair, retouch the roots only. Restraightening all of your hair can badly damage it.

- POOR DIET You can get the best haircut money can buy and use the richest conditioners, but it won't make a bit of difference if you don't have a well-balanced diet. A diet deficient in certain basic nutrients can take the shine right out of your hair, make it look lifeless and dull. To grow strong and healthy, your hair must be nourished from the roots up. Junk food might fill you up, but it's not good for your hair. Make sure to pack your diet with protein such as poultry, fish, and lean red meat. Eat lots of fresh fruits and vegetables and whole grains. And drink plenty of water. It's vital to your health and has no calories.

- LACK OF EXERCISE Poor circulation won't supply your hair with the nutrients it needs to stay glossy and healthy. You should exercise regularly—at least three times per week for twenty minutes at a time. Exercises designed to shape up certain spots on your body aren't enough. You have to get moving. Ride a bike, take a hike, go jogging. Your hair will love it.

• CHLORINE AND SALT WATER Hair that's been constantly exposed to salt water or chlorine can take on the consistency of straw. When you come out of the water, you've probably noticed that your skin feels drier. Well, the same thing is happening to your hair; you just can't feel it. Before you take the plunge, coat your hair with an instant conditioner. If you swim in a pool, wear a cap. After your swim, rinse your hair with fresh water, then shampoo and condition it. Finish with a vinegar rinse (see Chapter 7 on Sports Style) to remove any residue that might be trapped in the hair.

• STRESS When you're under stress (around exam time, for instance, or before an important sports competition), your oil glands will work overtime and may give you an attack of the greasies or aggravate a dandruff condition. Stress also makes you sweat, which can give your hair an unpleasant odor. In extreme cases, stress can even cause your hair to fall out. The remedies: a proper diet, plenty of sleep, and regular exercise, which helps relieve tension.

If you find it hard to unwind, deep-relaxation exercises can help. Here's one to try that really works. Lie down on your back on the floor, not on your bed; you don't want to get so comfortable that you fall asleep. Try to clear your mind of all worries. Imagine that you're floating on a cloud or lying on a raft in the middle of a blue sea. Start with your toes and relax them one by one. Then relax your feet, your ankles, your calves, your thighs. Next do your arms the same way, starting with your fingertips. Go on to your buttocks, your chest, your shoulders. Finish by relaxing your neck and head. Remain relaxed, concentrating only on pleasant thoughts for about ten minutes. When you're ready to come out of deep relaxation, take a few minutes to wake up your body slowly.

 ## COMMON HAIR WOES

If your hair sometimes looks dull and lifeless, and if it splits easily, you're not alone. These are problems that can afflict everyone. Here are the most common hair woes, their causes, and cures.

- SPLIT ENDS   Frazzled hair can be caused by too much heat, chemical processing, hard brushing, or a combination of all these things. Long hair is particularly prone to split ends, because scalp oils have farther to travel to reach the ends than they do in short hair. And once a split starts, it can travel all the way up the hairshaft. The only way to get rid of split ends is to cut them off, but this doesn't mean you have to cut your long hair short. Your hairdresser can just snip off the split ends. Conditioning can help make your hair look better by filling in the cracks in the hairshaft, but it will only work temporarily. No conditioner can actually cure split ends.
- HAIR BREAKAGE   Hair breakage is often mistaken for hair loss. Hair breakage can occur anywhere on the hairshaft; hair loss stems from the hair root it-

self. Breakage can be caused by overprocessing from perms, straightening, or coloring. Too much sun or overuse of styling appliances can also make your hair dry and brittle to the point of breakage. Hair that's in good condition is springy. If you pull a healthy hair taut, it will stretch and bounce back into shape. Brittle hair snaps off when you pull it because it has no elasticity. If breakage is your problem, avoid putting harsh chemicals on your hair. Wear it in a loose style. Give your hair a rest. Treat it gently, and step up your conditioning program.

- DRAB HAIR   It could be that you're not washing your hair enough. Choose a shampoo appropriate for your hair type, and wash your hair at the first sign of oiliness. Follow up with a light conditioner, and for maximum shine finish with a vinegar rinse (see page 132). Dullness can also be brought on by dryness, which can be caused by overprocessing or too much heat. If this is your problem, use a dry hair shampoo and deep condition your hair every two weeks with a thick cream conditioner. Brush your hair daily to get the oils flowing and to bring out shine. Also look to your eating habits for causes of dull hair. A poorly balanced diet could be the culprit.

- FINE FLYAWAY HAIR   Fine hair is something you're born with, but there are many ways to keep it under control. Static electricity can build up in fine hair, especially during the winter, causing your flyaway problem. To combat static electricity, use a shampoo containing protein, plus a body-building conditioner. Blowdrying will help fluff up fine limp hair. (Apply a setting lotion beforehand, to give your hair more body.) You might also want to consider a perm to give your hair more texture.

MORE SERIOUS PROBLEMS

Certain hair and scalp problems require immediate attention or they can get out of hand. Severe dandruff or a sudden and noticeable loss of hair can be the symptoms of more serious conditions which need to be treated by a doctor.

• DANDRUFF If you have dandruff, it's not the end of the world. Believe it or not, dandruff is an affliction that strikes almost everyone at one time or another. And contrary to common belief, it is not contagious. You can't get it by using someone else's comb or brush, or by sleeping on the same pillow as someone who has dandruff.

The primary symptom of dandruff is an itchy flaky scalp. The skin cells on the scalp are shed faster than normal, clumping together to form white flakes. These may cling to the scalp or fall onto your shoulders and back. There is another, more severe type of dandruff called *seborrheic dermatitis,* in which redness and inflammation accompany the scaling and itching. Red patches can appear on other parts of the body besides the scalp—on the sides of the nose, the area around the ears, and the center of the chest.

No one knows what causes dandruff, but during your teens, when your glands are pumping out more oil than ever, you may be more susceptible to it. The best way to treat it is with a specially formulated dandruff shampoo, and there are many good ones available. Wash your hair as often as you have to to control oiliness and scaling. Avoid greasy foods. Don't overbrush your hair. Try to stay calm—dandruff seems to flare up at times of stress. With this treatment, you should be able to get your dandruff under control in about a month. But if your dandruff persists, see a dermatologist—your scalp condition could be a sign of something more serious.

• COMBINATION HAIR   If your hair is oily or flaky on the scalp and parched on the ends, you have combination hair. This condition is often accompanied by oiliness or scales in the center of the forehead, on the sides of the nose or on the chest. Don't make the mistake of treating your hair as if it were too dry—you'll just aggravate the condition. But don't use a harsh shampoo made for oily hair or a strong dandruff formula, either—it will dry out the ends of the hair even more. The best way to treat combination hair is with a mild dandruff shampoo to control the oiliness or scaling and a conditioner applied to the ends of the hair only. You should also brush your hair daily to distribute oils from the scalp to the dry ends.

• HAIR LOSS   If you see many hairs coming out on your comb or brush, don't panic. It's normal to lose up to a hundred hairs per day. A sudden, severe loss of hair, however, is cause for concern. Stress, illness, medication, and dietary deficiencies can result in temporary hair loss. Pulling your hair back every day in a taut ponytail or braid, or sleeping with tightly wound rollers in your hair can result in a more serious type of hair loss—a receding hairline. If you think your hair is falling out at an abnormal rate, see a doctor.

 # QUESTIONS AND ANSWERS

Here are some of the questions asked most often about hair and its care.

1. *Will cutting my hair make it grow faster?*

The idea that cutting your hair will speed its growth is a myth. Healthy hair grows about half an inch per month. Split ends, however, can slow down the growth rate of your hair. The hair needs a steady supply of oxygen to grow, and split ends reduce the amount of oxygen that reaches the inside of the hairshaft. Have the split ends trimmed off, and your hair will grow at the normal rate once again.

2. *Why can't I use regular bath soap to wash my hair?*

Just because bath soap is mild enough for your skin doesn't mean that it's gentle on your hair. Human scalp and hair are naturally acidic, and washing your hair with a highly alkaline cleanser like bath soap can disrupt the natural acid mantle of your scalp, leaving your hair dry, rough, and limp. Bath soap creates lots of lather, which can make you think it's doing a great job of cleaning your hair. But these suds leave a dulling residue on the hair, even after a thorough rinsing. No matter how rushed you are, take the time to wash your hair with a shampoo that's formulated for your hair type, rather than reaching for a bar of soap.

3. *My hair looks coarse, but my hairdresser recently told me that it's really fine. How can this be true?*

It's often difficult to determine hair texture just by looking at or feeling the hair. You probably have thick fine hair, which makes it look coarse. The texture of your hair depends on the actual shape of the hair strands. Under a microscope, a cross section of fine hair looks flat; medium-textured hair is oval-shaped, and thick hair is round. Incidentally, hair color will determine how much hair you have. Blonds have the most hair—about 140,000 strands; brunets come in second with 110,000 strands; and redheads have the least amount of hair—about 90,000 strands.

4. *What's the difference between a home perm and a salon perm?*

The chemicals in a home perm solution are usually milder than those in the salon type—in case you use the product incorrectly. A salon perm generally contains conditioners the home perm does not. It stands to reason that you won't be as skilled as a professional stylist at giving yourself a perm, so if you want a problem-free perm that looks totally natural, your best bet is to go to a salon.

5. *I permed my slightly wavy, layered hair about four months ago and now that it's growing out, it's straighter at the crown than at the ends. Is there any way I can stretch out my perm for a few more months before I get another one?*

To perk up your perm, spray your hair with a light liquid setting lotion after you wash it. Setting lotion will give your hair more body and make the most of what's left of your perm. Let your hair dry naturally and fluff it up with your fingers. When it's almost dry, brush it lightly to blend in your natural waves with the permed curls. You can use setting lotion, or just mist your hair with water anytime your hair needs a lift.

6. *If I leave conditioner on my hair instead of washing it out, will it keep on working?*

All conditioners are designed to be rinsed out. They are effective only for as long as the package says. If you don't rinse out a conditioner, your hair will look dull and heavy. It's especially important to remove all traces of protein conditioners. If not completely rinsed out, they can leave a coating on the hair that flakes off during combing or brushing.

7. *I'm black and my hair is dry and difficult to comb. What's the proper way to care for it?*

Your problem is fairly common among black girls and women. Black hair looks tough, but it's really very fragile. It tends to be naturally dry and flyaway, and can break easily—especially if subjected to straightening, constant heat from blowdrying, or other abuse.

Choose a mild shampoo or one specially formulated for dry hair. There are also special shampoos available formulated for use on your hair. Wash your hair as often as necessary to keep it clean and fragrant, but be gentle. Apply a small amount of shampoo and work it evenly through from front to back, using the ends of your fingers—never your nails. One lathering is all you need unless your hair is very dirty. Don't scrub or pile your hair on top of your head—it can tangle easily. Follow up with a conditioner—a must if your hair has been straightened—and a vinegar rinse to smooth out the cuticle and impart a beautiful sheen. (See page 132 for an easy-to-make vinegar rinse.) Pat your hair dry with an absorbent towel and gently comb out the snarls. Use a wide-tooth comb to prevent breakage.

If you set your hair, avoid using sponge rollers. They can rob your hair of vital moisture and make it more susceptible to split ends and breakage. If you like to wear your hair in cornrows, you can leave them in for about a week and just shampoo your scalp. Make your braids loose to avoid unnecessary stress on the hair. Be sure to remove all ornaments from your cornrows before you go to bed at night for the same reason.

8. *I straightened my hair about a month ago, and now it's dry and dull. Will neutral henna restore its shine?*

Henna is one of the worst things you could put on your hair in its present condition. The straightening solution was probably left on your hair too long and dried it out, resulting in a lack of shine. Henna tends also to be drying and will only damage your hair more and may even cause breakage. So give your hair a rest. Try a hot oil treatment once or twice a week to restore moisture and smooth down the cuticle. Your hair will look more lustrous.

9. *I love the convenience of short hair, but would like to make it look different. What can I do?*

There are many things you can do to enhance short hair. Try tucking your hair behind your ears and slipping on a thin headband, or clip on some small colorful barrettes to hold the sides back. A bandanna tied on Indian-style looks pretty on short hair. If you have bangs, try brushing them back off your face, or create bangs where there weren't any before by combing the crown hair forward. For a sophisticated style, slick all of your hair back with a setting gel. Changing your part can make a big difference too. If you part your hair down the center, try a side part for a change. A body wave or soft perm is another option you might want to consider.

10. *I'm thinking of cutting my shoulder-length hair short, but I'm not sure whether I'd like it. Do you have any suggestions?*

If you're unsure about whether or not to cut your hair short, don't submit to the scissors until you've given it careful thought. You've invested a lot of time and care in growing your hair. A good compromise: Cut your hair gradually, a few inches more each time you visit the hairdresser. You might find that you like your hair at a certain length so much that you'll want to keep it that way and not go any shorter. You might also consider having your hair cut in graduated layers at the sides and bangs to add more interest.

ABOUT THE AUTHOR

Courtney DeWitt has worked for several national women's magazines and specializes in writing about fashion, beauty, and health. In her leisure time, she enjoys swimming and modern dance. She lives in New York City.

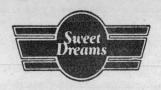

Read these great new *Sweet Dreams* romances, on sale soon:

☐ **#37 PORTRAIT OF LOVE by Jeanette Nobile (On sale April 15, 1983 • 23340-8 • $1.95)**
—Samantha's not sure she's going to like Santa Barbara—it doesn't have skyscrapers or the Yankees. However, it does have Tony Pappas, boy artist. But art is Tony's first love, and Samantha's mother is teaching him how to paint—the two of them spend hours talking and working together. Samantha feels like the odd man out. How can she get Tony's undivided attention?

☐ **#38 RUNNING MATES by Jocelyn Saal (On sale April 15, 1983 • 23341-6 • $1.95)**
—Carole and Steve were a couple once, but that seems like long ago. Yet now that they're both running for school president, Steve seems to be changing, opening up—and Carole finds herself falling in love again. What will happen when the votes are counted and only one is a winner?

☐ **#39 FIRST LOVE by Debra Spector (On sale May 15, 1983 • 23509-5 • $1.95)**
—Tracy and her mother agree—this is going to be Tracy's summer of romance. But mom wants her to date a worldly, sophisticated boy, while Tracy has her eye on David, the assistant chef at the restaurant where she works. He likes her too, and they'd be a perfect couple—if only Tracy's mother would give him a chance.

☐ **#40 SECRETS by Anna Aaron (On sale May 15, 1983 • 23510-9 •$1.95)**

—Ginny falls for Hal the first time she sees him. But though their dates are lots of fun, she can't tell how he really feels about her. And even after she lets his pet boa constrictor go for a stroll on her arm, Hal won't open up. Does he like her or doesn't he?

☐ **THE SWEET DREAMS BEAUTIFUL HAIR BOOK by Courtney DeWitt (On sale May 15, 1983 • 23375-0 • $1.95)**

—If your hair sometimes seems like your worst enemy, don't despair. Whether it's thick or thin, curly or straight, fine or coarse, blond or brunette—or somewhere in between—THE SWEET DREAMS BEAUTIFUL HAIR BOOK has all the secrets to help you stop fighting your hair—and start flaunting it.

Buy these books at your local bookstore or use this handy coupon for ordering: